The Complete Yoga Anatomy Coloring Book

of related interest

Yoga Teaching Handbook
Practical Guide for Yoga Teachers and Trainees
Edited by Sian O'Neill
ISBN 978 1 84819 355 0
eISBN 978 0 85701 313 2

Teen Yoga For Yoga Therapists
A Guide to Development, Mental Health and Working with Common Teen Issues
Charlotta Martinus
Foreword by Sir Anthony Seldon
ISBN 978 1 84819 399 4
eISBN 978 0 85701 355 2

Yoga Therapy for Fear
Treating Anxiety, Depression and Rage with the Vagus Nerve and Other Techniques
Beth Spindler with Kat Heagberg and Kevin Richardson
ISBN 978 1 84819 374 1
eISBN 978 0 85701 331 6

Principles and Themes in Yoga Therapy
An Introduction to Integrative Mind/Body Yoga Therapeutics
James Foulkes
Foreword by Mikhail Kogan, MD
Illustrated by Simon Barkworth
ISBN 978 1 84819 248 5
eISBN 978 0 85701 194 7

THE COMPLETE YOGA ANATOMY COLORING BOOK

KATIE LYNCH

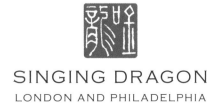

SINGING DRAGON
LONDON AND PHILADELPHIA

First published in 2019
by Singing Dragon
an imprint of Jessica Kingsley Publishers
73 Collier Street
London N1 9BE, UK
and
400 Market Street, Suite 400
Philadelphia, PA 19106, USA

www.singingdragon.com

Library of Congress Cataloging in Publication Data
A CIP catalog record for this book is available from the Library of Congress

British Library Cataloguing in Publication Data
A CIP catalogue record for this book is available from the British Library

ISBN 978 1 84819 420 5

Printed and bound in Great Britain by Bell and Bain Ltd, Glasgow

Contents

YOGA ANATOMY
INTRODUCTION

The best way to learn something is to internalize it. Much like having a strong foundation in yoga stems from getting to know the self, having a strong foundation in yoga anatomy stems from getting to know the body. As we work in asana, the mind–body connection strengthens and we begin to become aware of more structures inside our bodies. Muscles begin to contract and relax into our awareness and we start to become aware of the breath. As the perceptions of our bodies change, a natural curiosity about what our bodies are doing may arise. Learning the science behind the function of the body can bring a more holistic perspective that will further increase our understanding of the self.

Yoga anatomy benefits yogis in multiple ways. One way is to reinforce an already learned concept and another is to introduce a new concept. If a yogi becomes aware of his or her own iliopsoas during asana, learning the functions of the muscles can deepen the understanding of how the muscle works and can increase the control a yogi has over that muscle. Conversely, if a yogi does not feel his or her own iliopsoas in asana, learning the origin and insertion of the muscle can help the mind begin to imagine where the muscle would be, what it would look like, and how it would function in certain poses. This way of learning can eventually create a mind–body connection with the structure that can lead to voluntary control over the iliopsoas.

As you color, bringing your mind to your own body can help bring awareness and reinforce concepts. Try to feel and internalize the muscle or structure in your own body. When you're coloring the abductors of the thighs, think about poses that require these muscles. Get up to move and feel how the abductors contract. Allowing the mind and body to learn together will trigger kinesthetic learning and further deepen the mind–body connection. The stronger your connection is with the body, the stronger your awareness is of the world.

PART I
ANATOMY

ANATOMY TERMS

In anatomy, directional terms describe the location of structures inside the body. Anatomical terms refer to a body that is in the anatomical position. This way the direction cannot be mistaken. The anatomical position is the same position as tadasana (mountain pose) with the palms facing forwards. The reference is from the inside of the body, as if you are the person in the anatomical position talking about your right or left sides of the body.

Anterior: a direction that refers to the front side of a body. *Example:* the pectoralis major is located on the anterior side of the body.

Posterior: a direction that refers to the back side of a body. *Example:* the gluteus maximus is located on the posterior side of the body.

Superior: a direction that refers to something above, towards the head. *Example:* the heart is superior to the ovaries.

Inferior: a direction that refers to something below, towards the feet. *Example:* the knee joint is inferior to the hip joint.

Lateral: a direction that refers to something further away from the midline of the body. *Example:* the arms are lateral to the spine.

Medial: a direction that refers to something closer to the midline of the body. *Example:* the sacrum is medial to the head of the femur bone.

Proximal: a direction that refers to something closer to the limb's attachment to the trunk. *Example:* the femur is proximal to the fibula.

Distal: a direction that refers to something further away from the limb's attachment to the trunk. *Example:* the ulna is distal to the humerus.

Deep: a direction that refers to something further in from the surface of the body. *Example:* the pectoralis minor is deep to the pectoralis major.

Superficial: a direction that refers to something closer to the surface of the body. *Example:* the gluteus medius is superficial to the gluteus minimus.

BONES INTRODUCTION

During childhood, the skeleton consists of around 270 bones. Once the skeleton has reached adulthood and some bones have fused together, the skeleton is left with 206 bones. The bones of the skeleton are the internal frameworks of the human body. They allow our bodies to walk upright and move in a variety of different ways. When two or more bones come together to meet another bone, this point of connection becomes a joint. Joints allow the skeleton to move, and the muscles provide stabilization for the joints and create the movements of the joints.

There are many types of textures that exist on human bones. The surface of a bone consists of projections, fissures, ridges, grooves, protuberances, and other features that indicate a unique connection with another structure of the human body. Every bone is unique, and the markings can tell what ligaments, tendons, blood vessels, or nerves attach to or run through the bone. Familiarizing yourself with the surfaces of bones can help give a deeper understanding of how the muscles attach to the bones.

MUSCLES INTRODUCTION

Many muscles work on a voluntary and involuntary level. They can function without us telling them to do so or we can take control of our muscles to bring our bodies into a more conscious movement. Learning about how the muscles function will help increase conscious control over the muscles in the body.

Each muscle has an origin, insertion, and an action(s). As a muscle contracts, there are agonistic and antagonistic muscles that work to help a muscle function more efficiently.

Origin: skeletal muscles have tendons and those tendons attach to bone. An origin is the place of attachment for a muscle. It is where the muscle originates. The origin of a muscle is commonly a fixed place of attachment.

Insertion: an insertion is also a place of attachment for a muscle and is commonly attached to a bone that moves with contraction.

Muscles span across joints in order to move bones. For example, the biceps brachii's primary movement is elbow flexion. In order to flex the elbow, the muscle originates across the shoulder joint, runs down the humerus, and spans across the elbow joint to attach to the radius bone of the forearm. This way, when the biceps muscle contracts, it will shorten and pull the forearm up towards the shoulder joint to produce flexion of the elbow. Similar to the biceps brachii, many muscles cross over more than one joint and are capable of moving more than one structure. When the origins and insertions of muscles are understood, the mystery of how the body moves begins to unfold.

Agonists: muscles that are primarily responsible for controlling a specific movement. Also referred to as prime movers.

Antagonists: muscles that oppose prime movers.

In the body, there are agonistic and antagonistic pairs of muscles or muscle groups. For example, when the hamstrings contract, the quadriceps lengthen. And conversely, when the hamstrings lengthen, the quadriceps contract. An antagonistic muscle lengthens while the agonistic muscle contracts in order to assist the prime mover (agonist group) in action. If the hamstrings did not lengthen while the quadriceps contracted, it would take much more force to contract the quadriceps and the body would have to spend more energy to move.

Learning about how the muscles move individually and how they work together will help you zone in on areas of your own body that may have imbalances due to postural behaviors. Knowing about your own imbalances will make it easier to figure out what movements need to be done in order to restore balance to your body.

MUSCLE MOVEMENTS

The body can be broken down into movements. Movements are often paired with opposing movements and each occurs on the opposite side of the joint being moved. For example, the hip flexors contract to flex the hip, while the hip extensors contract to extend the hip. The hip flexor muscles are located on the anterior side of the hip joint, while the hip extensor muscles are located on the posterior side of the hip joint. Get to know the movement terms of the body and think about which limbs might perform each movement.

Abduction: the movement of a limb or structure laterally from the midline of the body.

Adduction: the movement of a limb or structure medially towards the midline of the body.

Flexion: a movement that decreases the angle between two bones.

Extension: a movement that increases the angle between two bones.

Internal rotation: a movement that rotates a limb inward towards the midline of the body.

External rotation: a movement that rotates a limb away from the midline of the body.

Depression: a movement that refers to the shoulder blades sliding inferiorly.

Elevation: a movement that refers to the shoulder blades raising superiorly.

Protraction: a movement that refers to the shoulder blades laterally moving away from the midline.

Retraction: a movement that refers to the shoulder blades medially moving towards the midline.

Upward rotation: a movement that rotates the inferior angle of the scapula superiorly and laterally.

Downward rotation: a movement that rotates the inferior angle of the scapula inferiorly and medially towards the midline of the body.

Pronation: a movement that rotates the forearm so that the palms face backwards.

Supination: a movement that rotates the forearm so that the palms face forwards.

Dorsiflexion: the flexion of the ankle joint that brings the toes upwards towards the shin.

Plantar flexion: the extension of the ankle joint that points the toes downwards.

Inversion: a movement that tilts the sole of the foot inward towards the midline.

Eversion: a movement that tilts the sole of the foot outward away from the midline.

Lateral flexion: a movement that bends the spine laterally away from the midline of the body.

Circumduction: the circular movement of the limb. A combination of flexion, extension, adduction, and abduction.

Rotation: a movement that rotates around an axis.

STRUCTURE OF A SKELETAL MUSCLE

The structure of a skeletal muscle is made up of contractile threads, muscle fibers, layers of fascia, blood vessels, and nerve endings (motor neurons). The tiny fibers of a muscle are the muscle's cells. They are grouped together and wrapped in a dense fibrous connective tissue known as fascia. The groups of fibers are then bundled together and wrapped in more fascia. When the fascia wraps the last group of bundles, an entire muscle is formed. Fascia wraps around layers of muscle fibers to reduce friction with surrounding muscles or bones. Tendons form on each muscle and attach muscles to bones. Blood vessels are interwoven throughout the muscle for blood supply, and nerve endings run through the muscle for mind–body communication. The structure of a skeletal muscle is broken down into: myofibrils, muscle fibers, endomysium, muscle fascicles, perimysium, and epimysium.

Myofibrils: thin and thick threads found in muscle cells that are responsible for muscular contractions (actin and myosin).

Muscle fibers (cells): muscle cells in the shape of long fibers containing myofibrils.

Endomysium: a thin layer of areolar connective tissue that wraps individual muscle fibers (muscle cells). The endomysium also contains capillaries and nerves.

Muscle fascicles: a bundle of skeletal muscle fibers wrapped in perimysium. Each bundle contains 10–100 muscle fibers.

Perimysium: a sheath of connective tissue that wraps around muscle fascicles.

Epimysium: the outer layer of dense connective tissue that surrounds an entire skeletal muscle and reduces friction between muscles or surrounding bones.

STRUCTURE OF A SKELETAL MUSCLE

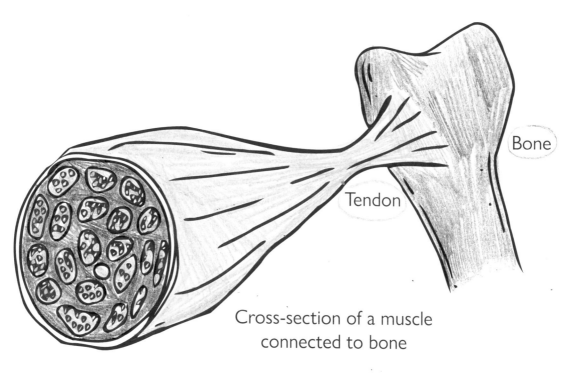

Bone

Tendon

Cross-section of a muscle
connected to bone

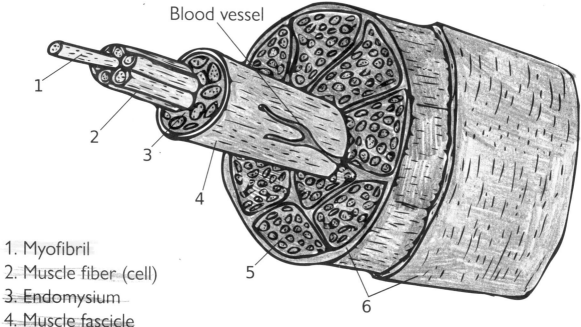

Blood vessel

1
2
3
4
5
6

1. Myofibril
2. Muscle fiber (cell)
3. Endomysium
4. Muscle fascicle
5. Perimysium
6. Epimysium

Cross-section of a
muscle zoomed in

MUSCLE CONTRACTION

Once the brain sends a signal to the muscle cell that it wants it to contract, the tubular myofibrils inside of a muscle cell perform a contraction process within a sarcomere. A sarcomere is the contractile and repeating unit within a myofibril. The myofibril consists of contractile threads of thin and thick proteins called actin and myosin. Actin protein filaments are thin, and myosin protein filaments are thick. During contraction, the actin and myosin filaments slide over one another causing the length of the sarcomere to shorten. Zones of importance are labeled on the sarcomere.

A-band: an A-band contains the entire length of the thick myosin filaments. This area does not change length during contraction.

H-zone: a subdivision within the A-band. In this zone, there are only thick myosin protein filaments present. This area shortens during muscle contraction as the filaments slide over each other.

M-line: a line within the middle of the H-zone and sarcomere.

I-band: an area within the sarcomere that contains only thin actin protein filaments. This area shortens during muscle contraction.

Z-line: the border of the sarcomere, composed of actin molecules. As the muscle contracts, the Z-lines are brought closer together.

MUSCLE CONTRACTION

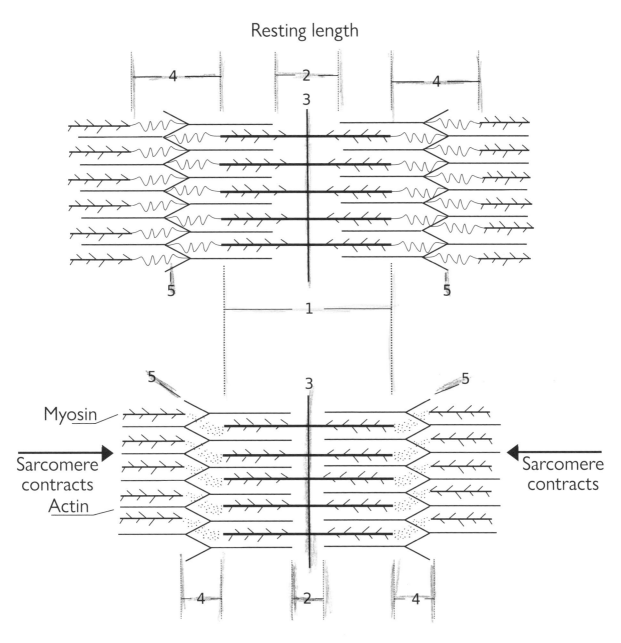

Resting length

Myosin

Sarcomere
contracts
Actin

Sarcomere
contracts

Contracted

1. A-band
2. H-zone
3. M-line
4. I-band
5. Z-line

JOINT TYPES

A joint is the site of connection and attachment between separate bones for the purpose of movement. A synovial joint is made up of fibrous connective tissue, cartilage, and synovial fluid (lubrication). There are six types of synovial joints in the human body: pivot joints, plane joints, hinge joints, ball-and-socket joints, saddle joints, and ellipsoid joints.

Pivot joint: a joint that produces a rotary movement around a single axis. Pivot joints are seen when examining the radius and ulna connection. The radius and ulna create a rotary movement around each other during pronation and supination of the forearm. Pivot joints are also seen in the cervical spine when the head turns right and left.

Plane joint: also known as a gliding joint, a plane joint is a joint formed between bones with flat surfaces. During movement, plane joints glide against each other to produce movement. Plane joints are seen when examining some of the bones in the ankles and the wrists.

Hinge joint: a joint that moves two bones along one axis to extend or flex. Examples of a hinge joint include the elbow joint and knee joint, which produce flexion and extension.

Ball-and-socket joint: a joint that consists of a bone with a ball-shaped surface that fits into a cup-like depression of another bone. This arrangement gives rise to a joint with a wide range of movement. Two major ball-and-socket joints in the human body are the hip joint and the glenohumeral joint of the shoulder.

Saddle joint: a joint that consists of one bone shaped like a saddle and another bone that fits into the shape of the saddle. The first metacarpal of the thumb forms a saddle joint with the trapezium bone of the wrist.

Ellipsoid joint: also referred to as a condyloid joint, an ellipsoid joint consists of an oval bone that fits into an elliptical cavity. Ellipsoid joints allow for flexion, extension, adduction, abduction, and circumduction. The bones of the wrist consist of bones that create ellipsoidal joints.

JOINT TYPES

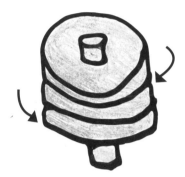

Pivot joint

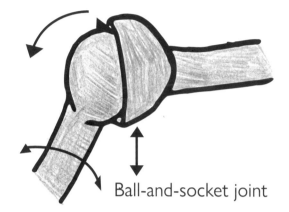

Ball-and-socket joint

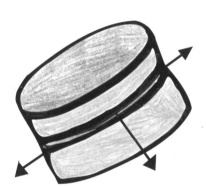

Plane joint

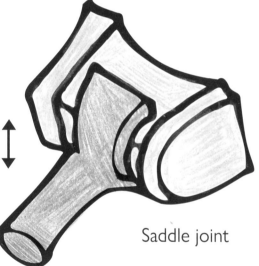

Saddle joint

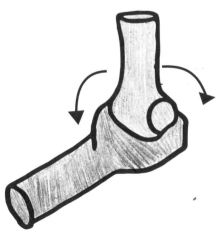

Hinge joint

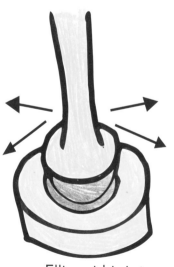

Ellipsoid joint

THE SPINE

The spine consists of 24 individual vertebrae that provide support and protection to the skeletal and nervous system. Nerves from the brain run down the spinal column and branch out to form the peripheral nervous system. The peripheral nerves connect to muscles and transmit communication from the brain to tell the muscles to contract or relax. The spine is broken down into five sections: the cervical spine (C1–C7), the thoracic spine (T1–T12), the lumbar spine (L1–L5), the sacrum (S1–S5), and the coccyx (Co1–Co4). The cervical spine and lumbar spine form a curve of lordosis (concave curve), and the thoracic spine and sacrum form a curve called kyphosis (convex curve). Tiny muscles and ligaments run along the spaces of the vertebrae to knit and stabilize the spine, while larger muscles run the length of the spine to support the spine during movement. When the muscles around the spine contract, they bring the spine into flexion, extension, lateral flexion, and rotation. Weak muscles of the spine or poor postural behaviors can bring the spine out of alignment. Misalignments put unhealthy strain onto the spine and can cause discomfort and increase the chances of injury. In order to keep the spine aligned and healthy, yoga poses that put the spine through the range of movements it can produce can work to bring the spine into alignment and can decrease strain and chances of injury.

Cervical vertebrae: the cervical spine consists of the first seven vertebrae of the spine and make up the neck. When aligned, the cervical vertebrae form a curve of lordosis. The cervical spine can flex, extend, rotate, and laterally flex without the movement of the lower portion of the spine. The cervical vertebrae are smaller in size than the rest of the vertebrae. The first and second cervical vertebrae (C1–C2) are referred to as atlas and axis. Atlas does not have a vertebral body and is fused with axis. Together they form the joint that connects the spine to the skull and have a wide range of lateral motion. The seventh cervical vertebra (C7) has the largest spinous process and can be palpated.

Thoracic vertebrae: the thoracic spine contains 12 vertebrae (T1–T12) and starts when the spine begins a kyphosis curve after C7. The transverse process of each vertebra connects to a set of ribs, which together form the ribcage.

Lumbar vertebrae: the lumbar vertebrae consist of five large vertebrae (L1–L5) and make up the lodorsis curve of the lower back. The lumbar spine supports the majority of the weight in the spine and connects to the sacrum. Since the lumbar spine is capable of carrying weight, it can often become strained if too much weight is put onto it. Strain in the lumbar spine causes lower back pain and can damage ligaments, muscles, or the discs between the vertebrae.

Sacrum: the sacrum is a wedge-shaped vertebra that is located at the end of the spine and sits in between the two hipbones. Together, the two hipbones and the sacrum articulate and form the two sacroiliac joints (SI joints). The sacroiliac joints are held in place by ligaments and muscles and have very little room for movement. The sacrum takes the weight from the spine and transfers it to the hipbones. The sacrum fuses after adolescence and can be broken up into five vertebrae (S1–S5).

Coccyx: the coccyx is a small bone attached to the end of the sacrum and is the last bone to make up the vertebral column. Also known as the tailbone, the coccyx bone can be broken down into four tiny fused vertebrae (Co1–Co4).

THE SPINE

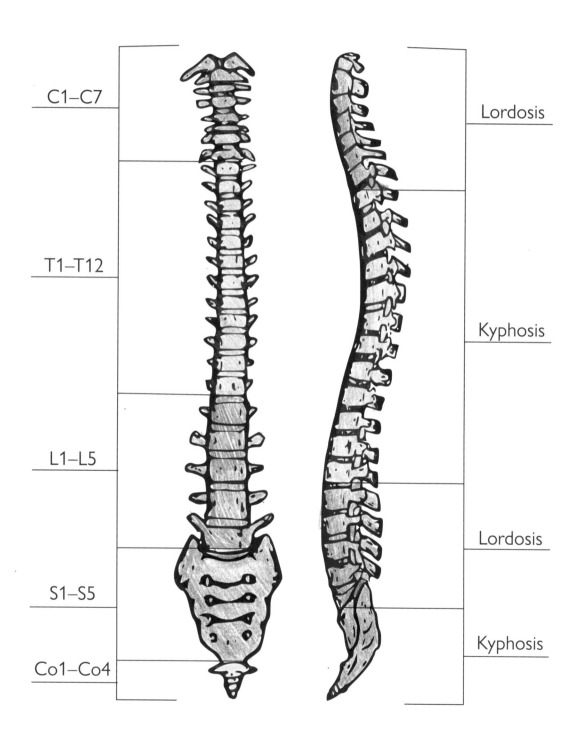

C1–C7

T1–T12

L1–L5

S1–S5

Co1–Co4

Lordosis

Kyphosis

Lordosis

Kyphosis

SPINAL VERTEBRAE

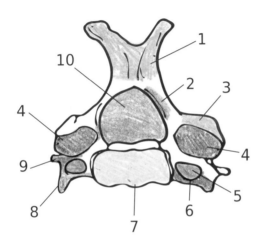

Cervicle Vertebrae
1. Spinous process
2. Lamina
3. Inferior articular process
4. Superior articular facet
5. Transverse foramen
6. Transverse process
7. Body
8. Anterior tubercle
9. Posterior tubercle
10. Vertebral foramen

Thoracic Vertebrae
1a. Spinous process
2a. Angle of articular facet
3a. Transverse costal facet
4a. Pedicle
5a. Superior costal facet
6a. Body
7a. Superior articular facet
8a. Lamina

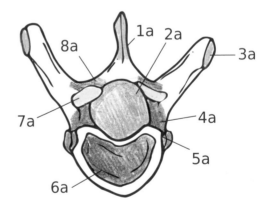

SPINAL VERTEBRAE

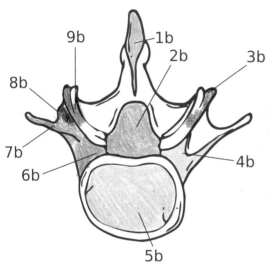

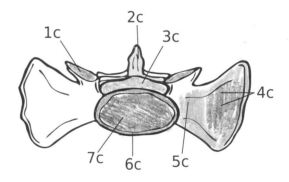

Lumbar Vertebrae
1b. Spinous process
2b. Vertebral foramen
3b. Mamillary process
4b. Pedicle
5b. Vertebral body
6b. Lamina
7b. Transverse process
8b. Accessory process
9b. Superior articular process

Sacrum
1c. Superior articular process
2c. Median sacral crest
3c. Sacral canal
4c. Lateral part of sacrum
5c. Wing of sacrum
6c. Promontory
7c. Base of sacrum

NECK MUSCLES

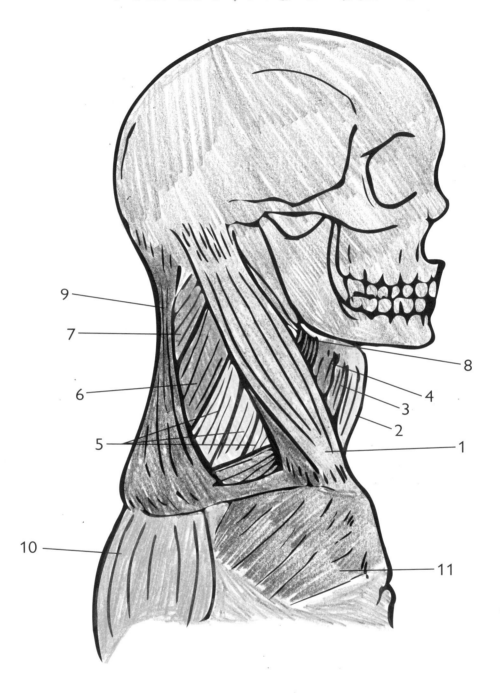

1. Steinocleidomastoid
2. Sternohyoid
3. Omohyoid
4. Thyrohyoid
5. Scalene muscles
6. Levator scapulae

7. Spenius capitus
8. Longus capitus
9. Trapezius
10. Deltoid
11. Pectoralis major

SPINAL MOVEMENTS

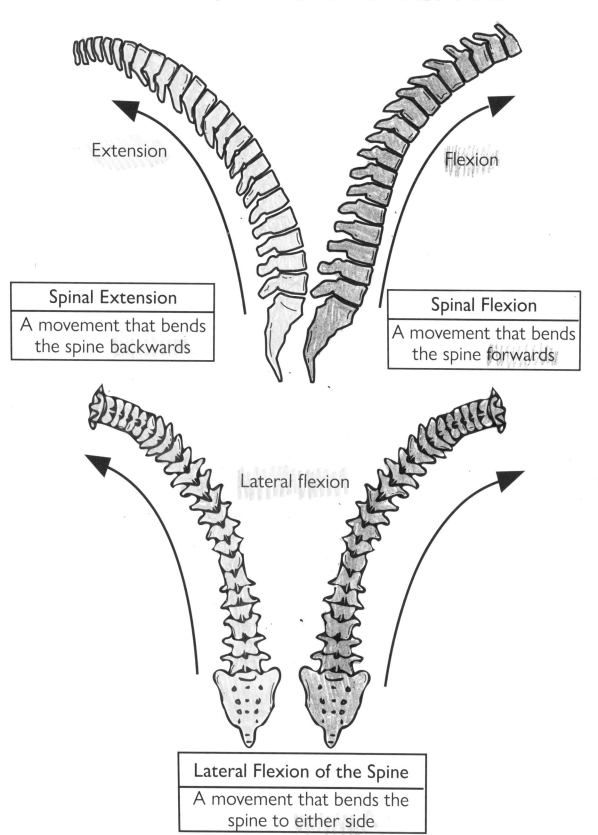

Extension

Flexion

Spinal Extension
A movement that bends the spine **backwards**

Spinal Flexion
A movement that bends the spine **forwards**

Lateral flexion

Lateral Flexion of the Spine
A movement that bends the spine to either side

SPINAL EXTENSORS

The spinal extensors are a group of muscles that contract to bend the spine backwards into extension. The muscles that create this movement are the erector spinae. The erector spinae are a set of muscles that contain the iliocostalis, longissimus, and spinalis. They run from the lumbar vertebrae to the base of the skull, running along both sides of the vertebral column. Tight spinal extensors can create lumbar pains, which can limit mobility. When working with the spine, or any part of the body, it is important to be gentle. Bring your awareness to the spine and stop at any sign of discomfort. To lengthen tight spinal extensors, yoga poses or movements that bring the spine into flexion begin to bring length to the muscles. Uttanasana (standing forwards fold) with knees bent and marjaryasana (cat pose) are some gentle yoga poses that bring the spine into flexion. In order to bring strength to the spinal extensors, yoga poses or movements that bring the spine into extension can bring strength to the muscles. Salambhasana (locust pose) and ustrasana (camel pose) work to bring strength to the spinal extensors.

To activate the spinal extensors

Lie on your stomach with your arms pressing into your side (adduction). Stabilize the lower half of your body by activating your core and pressing your hips, shins, and ankles into the ground. On an inhale, lift your chest and arms off the ground and hold for 10–30 seconds. Keep your breath relaxed. As you hold, energetically lengthen the spine towards your head and gaze at the ground in front of you to keep the neck from over extending. Release hold and rest for 10–30 seconds. Repeat 3–5 times.

What did you notice? Did you feel any muscles on your posterior side contracting? Did any areas feel unusually tense or overworked? Make a mental or physical note of your experience in order to get to know how your body is working. Practicing this exercise daily will help the spinal extensors bring strength and support to the spine during everyday movements.

SPINAL EXTENSORS

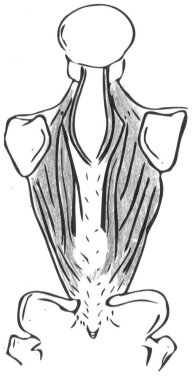

Erector spinae

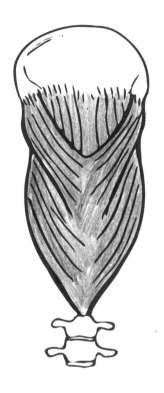

Splenius capitus, splenius
cervicis, semispinalis capitus

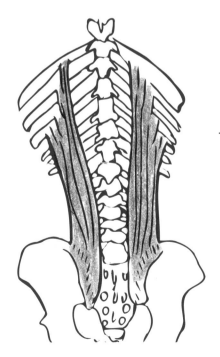

Iliocostalis

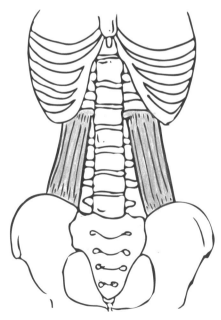

Quadratus lumborum

SPINAL FLEXORS

The spinal flexors are a group of muscles that bring the spine into a forwards bend. These muscles include the rectus abdominis and the iliopsoas. The transversus abdominis also plays a large role in compressing the abdominal contents in the abdominal cavity. As the transversus abdominis contracts to compress the abdomen, the spinal flexors are able to bring a stronger and more stable contraction to the spine. Tight spinal flexors can limit the spine's ability to extend. Yoga poses that bring the spine into extension will bring length to these muscles. Salabhasana (locust pose), salamba bhujangasana (sphinx pose) and dhanurasana (bow pose) are poses that bring length to the spinal flexors. If the spinal flexors are weak, back pain can arise as well.

Without strong support from the front of the spine, the body is more prone to injury during movement. Bringing the spine into flexion will help strengthen the flexors of the spine. Marjaryasana (cat pose) and kumbhakasana (plank pose) will help bring strength to the spinal flexors.

To activate the spinal flexors

Start on your hands and knees with your spine in a neutral alignment. Grab a folded blanket if your knees need cushion. Align your shoulders with your wrists and your hips with your knees. Press your shins and ankles into the ground for stability. On an exhale, lift or flex your spine towards the ceiling by slightly tucking your pelvis and activating your abdominals to move and support the spine into a flexed position (marjaryasana, cat pose). Draw your chin into your chest. Hold this position for 10–30 seconds then bring the spine back into a neutral position. Repeat 3–5 times.

What did you notice? Did you feel your abdominals contracting as your spine flexed and rounded towards the ceiling? Make a mental or physical note of what you felt. Practicing this exercise daily will help the muscles on the anterior spine strengthen and activate to bring support to the spine during movement.

SPINAL FLEXORS

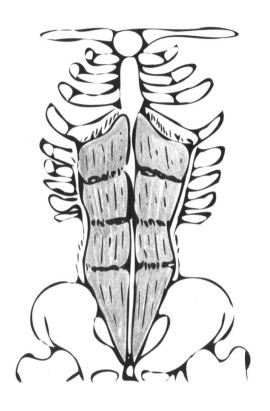

Rectus abdominis

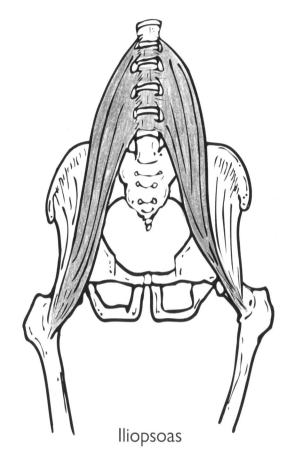

Iliopsoas

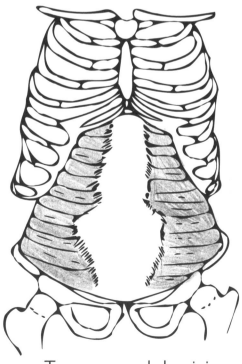

Transversus abdominis

LATERAL FLEXORS OF THE SPINE

The lateral flexors of the spine are a group of muscles that bring the spine into a side bending movement. The lateral flexors run along the right and left sides of the spine, and while one side of the lateral flexors contracts, the opposing side works as an antagonist and lengthens. The muscles responsible for lateral flexion of the spine are: the internal oblique, the external oblique, the rectus abdominis, the iliopsoas, the quadratus lumborum, the iliocostalis, the erector spinae, and the latissimus dorsi. Tight or weak lateral flexors inhibit the spine's ability to produce lateral flexion. Yoga poses that produce lateral flexion of the spine will help lengthen and strengthen the lateral flexors. Parsva urdhva hastasana (upward salute side bend pose) and parighasana (gate pose) are poses that bring length and strength to the lateral flexors of the spine.

To activate the lateral flexors

Start in mountain pose with your arms down by your side. Press your feet into the floor and stabilize your pelvis. Slightly activate the core to keep the ribcage from jutting out forwards. Energetically lengthen your spine towards your head. Relax your neck. On an inhale, abduct your arms out to the side to bring them overhead. On an exhale, laterally bend or flex the spine to the left. Hold this position for 5–10 seconds and then bring your spine back to a neutral position. Repeat the movement for the right side. Practice both movements 3–5 times.

What did you notice? Did the movement feel awkward and stiff? Or did it feel smooth and supported?

Lateral flexion of the spine is not a large movement and can be felt by shifting your ribcage to the right or left. As your spine laterally flexes, lengthen the spine in order to bring space to the vertebrae. This exercise can be done sitting in a chair, on the ground, or while standing. Practicing this exercise daily will help strengthen and activate the lateral flexors, which will help support the spine during everyday movements.

LATERAL FLEXORS
OF THE SPINE

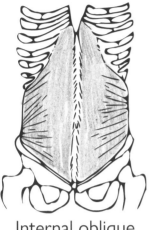

Internal oblique

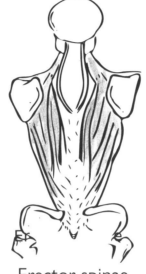

Erector spinae

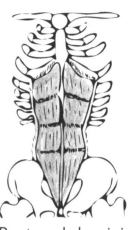

Rectus abdominis

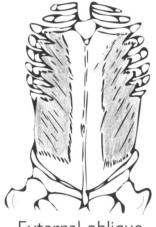

External oblique

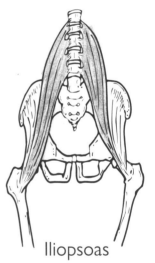

Iliopsoas

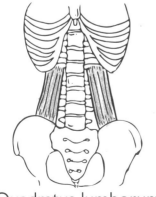

Quadratus lumborum

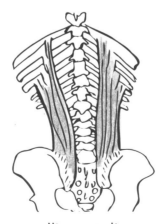

Iliocostalis

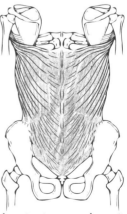

Latissimus dorsi

THE ABDOMINALS

The abdominals are a group of muscles that contract to bring movement to the spine. The abdominal group consists of four muscles: the transversus abdominis, the internal oblique, the external oblique, and the rectus abdominis. The four muscles also compress the abdominal contents in order to help the spine flex with ease and strength. Since the abdominals stabilize the pelvis and spine, when they become weak, the body's ability to balance during movement decreases. For example, when the body goes from sitting to standing, the abdominals activate to flex and balance the spine. If the abdominals are too weak to activate, the spine is unable to balance and the body will struggle. Weak abdominals can increase the chances of spinal injuries. To bring strength to the abdominals, yoga poses or movements that bring the spine into flexion will strengthen the muscles. Yoga poses like marjaryasana (cat pose) and navasana (boat pose) flex the spine and require the abdominals to contract. To lengthen tight abdominals, poses like bitilasana (cow pose) and urdhva dhanurasana (wheel pose) require the spine to extend and the abdominals to lengthen.

Transversus abdominis: the transversus abdominis is the deepest layer of the abdominals. When contracted, the muscles assist with lateral flexion of the spine. Since the transversus abdominis is the deepest layer, it plays a large role in compressing the contents of the abdominal cavity. Coupled with the contraction of the pelvic floor muscles, the transversus abdominis brings strength and balance to the spine when in inverted poses.

Internal oblique: the internal oblique originates from the seventh to twelfth costal cartilages of the ribs, thoracolumbar fascia, iliac crest, anterior superior iliac spine, and the iliopsoas fascia. The fibers run medially to insert onto the tenth to twelfth ribs and the linea alba. The internal oblique muscles contract to produce lateral flexion, rotation, and flexion of the trunk. They help the spine come into flexion with ease by compressing the abdominal contents in the abdominal cavity.

External oblique: the external oblique is the most superficial muscle of the group. It originates on the surfaces of the fifth to twelfth ribs. The fibers run medially and posteriorly and insert onto the linea alba, pubic tubercle, and anterior iliac crest. When the fibers contract, they bring the spine into flexion, lateral flexion, and assist with spinal rotation. During spinal flexion, the external oblique compresses the abdominal cavity and pulls the chest downwards.

Rectus abdominis: the rectus abdominis is the muscle known as the "six pack." It runs vertically on either side of the midline of the anterior trunk. It originates on the pubis of the pelvis and extends superiorly to insert onto the fifth to seventh rib cartilages and the xyphoid process of the sternum. When the fibers contract, the spine is brought into flexion. It compresses the contents of the abdomen and stabilizes the pelvis. The rectus abdominis also works to protect the spine from hyperextending during deep spinal extension poses.

TRANSVERSUS ABDOMINIS

Action: Compresses abdomen, unilaterally rotates trunk to same side

Origin: 7th–12th costal cartilages, thoracolumbar fascia, iliac crest, anterior iliac spine, iliopsoas fascia

Insertion: Linea alba, pubic crest

Agonists: Rectus abdominis, external/internal obliques

Antagonists: Erector spinae

Poses: *Contracts:* tadasana, marjaryasana, bakasana. *Lengthens:* parsvakonasana

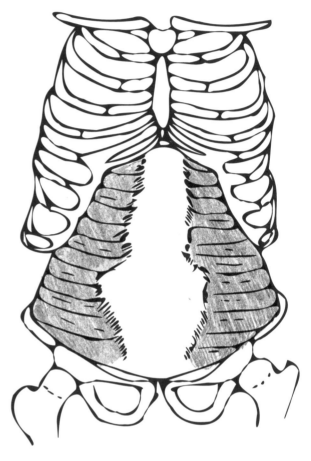

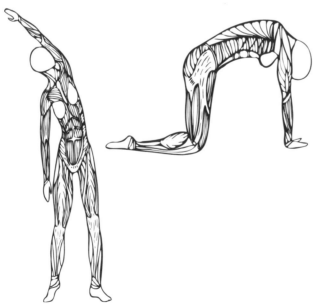

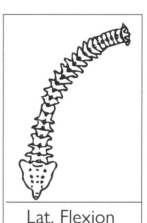

Lat. Flexion

INTERNAL OBLIQUE

Action: Lateral flexion of spine, rotation of spine. Flexion of trunk, compression of abdomen, and stabilization of pelvis

Origin: 7th–12th costal cartilages, thoracolumbar fascia, iliac crest, anterior superior iliac spine, iliopsoas fascia

Insertion: 10th–12th ribs, linea alba

Agonists: Rectus femoris, transversus abdominis, iliocostalis, longissimus, external oblique

Antagonists: Iliocostalis, longissimus, psoas major, external oblique

Poses: *Contracts and lengthens:* parighasana, utthita parsvakonasana, parsva urdhva hastasana

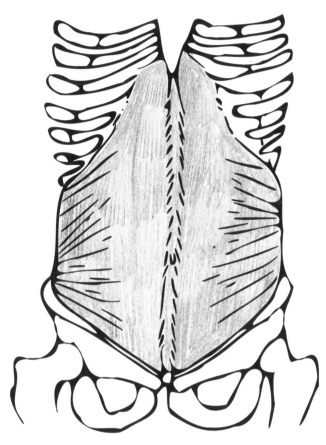

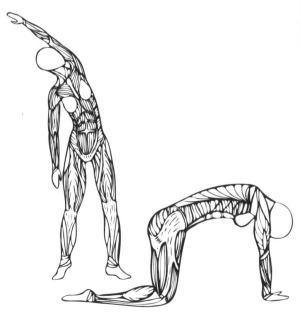

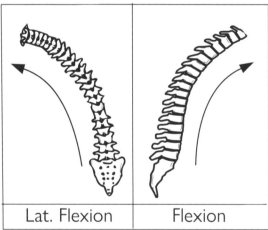

| Lat. Flexion | Flexion |

EXTERNAL OBLIQUE

Action: Lateral flexion of spine, flexes trunk, compresses abdomen, and stabilizes pelvis

Origin: 5th–12th ribs

Insertion: Linea alba, pubic tubercle, anterior iliac crest.

Agonists: *Lateral flexion:* erector spinae, internal obliques. *Flexion:* rectus abdominis, transversus abdominis

Antagonists: *Lateral flexion:* erector spinae, internal obliques (opposing side)

Poses: *Contracts and lengthens:* parsva urdhva hastasana, utthita parsvakonasana, ardha parsvottanasana

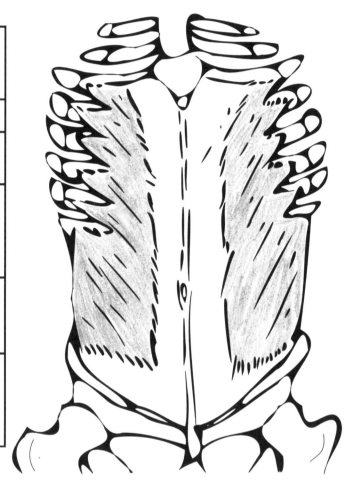

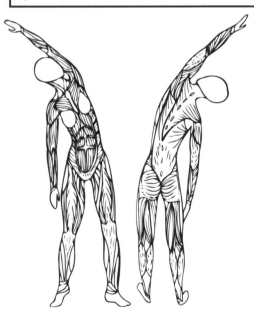

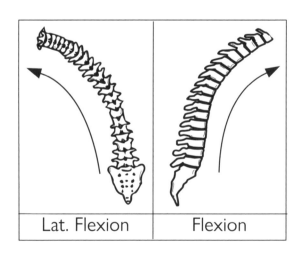

Lat. Flexion | Flexion

RECTUS ABDOMINIS

Action: Flexes the trunk, stabilizes the pelvis, and compresses the abdomen

Origin: Pubis

Insertion: 5th–7th rib cartilages, xiphoid process of sternum

Agonists: External/internal obliques, transversus abdominis

Antagonists: Iliocostalis, longissimus, spinalis, semispinalis

Poses: *Contracts:* marjaryasana, bakasana, navasana. *Lengthens:* bitilasana, ustrasana, urdhva dhanurasana

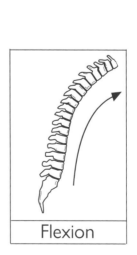

Flexion

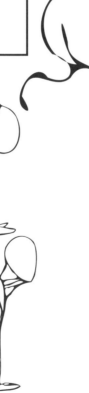

ERECTOR SPINAE

The erector spinae are a group of long, thin muscles that contract to bring the full spine into extension. The erector spinae can be broken down into three groups: the spinalis group, the longissimus group, and the iliocostalis group. The spinalis group and the longissimus group extend and rotate the head. The longissimus and iliocostalis group extend and laterally flex the spine. The erector spinae extend from the cervical spine, down the vertebral column, and on to the crest of the sacrum. Tight erector spinae can develop if the posture of the body favors spinal extension. The muscles can stiffen from over-activation and can cause discomfort. To lengthen the erector spinae, yoga poses or movements that bring the spine into flexion will elongate the muscles of extension. Some yoga poses that lengthen the erector spinae are marjaryasana (cat pose) and uttanasana (standing forwards fold). If the erector spinae muscles become weak from lack of extension, the ability to stabilize and support the spine during movement decreases. This can increase the chance of injury to the back, especially during poses with deep spinal extension. To strengthen the erector spinae, yoga poses or movements that bring the spine into extension, without putting too much weight onto the spine, will begin to strengthen the erector spinae and prepare the muscles of extension for more weight-bearing poses. Some yoga poses that bring strength to the erector spinae without putting too much weight onto the spine are salambhasana (locust pose) and bitilasana (cow pose).

ERECTOR SPINAE

Action: Extension and lateral flexion of spine (iliocostalis and longissimus). Extension and lateral flexion of cervicle and thoracic spine (spinalis)

Origin: C5–L3 spinous processes (spinalis). C4–T6 transverse processes, sacrum iliac crest (longissimus). 3rd–12th ribs, sacrum, iliac crest, thoracolumbar fascia (iliocostalis)

Insertion: C2–T8 spinous processes (spinalis). Temporal bone, C2–C5 transverse process, 2nd–12th ribs (longissimus), C4–C6 transverse process, 1st–6th ribs, thoracolumbar fascia (iliocostalis)

Agonists: Longissimus, spinalis, iliocostalis

Antagonists: *Extension:* rectus abdominis, external/internal obliques, transversus abdominis. *Lateral flexion:* opposing side muscles

Poses: *Contracts:* bitilasana, ustrasana, urdhva dhanurasana, salambhasana. *Lengthens:* marjaryasana, balasana, pashimottanasana

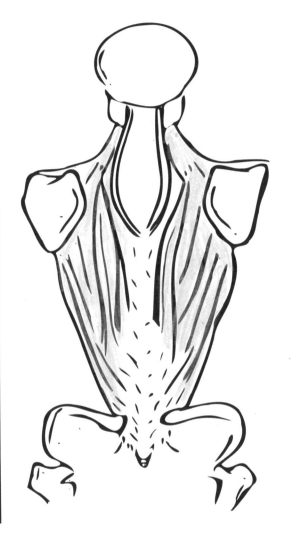

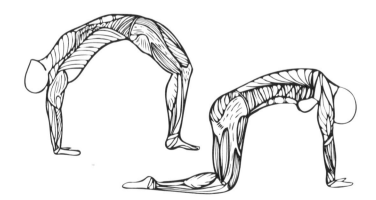

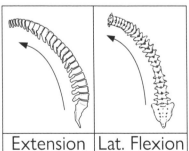

Extension | Lat. Flexion

ILIOCOSTALIS

The iliocostalis muscle runs on either side of the spine, extending from the posterior hipbones to the lateral ribcage. It is a part of the erector spinae group and contracts to extend and laterally flex the spine. It originates on the third to seventh ribs, sacrum, iliac crest, and thoracolumbar fascia. It extends upwards and inserts onto the C4–C6 vertebrae, first to sixth ribs, twelfth rib, and upper lumbar vertebrae.

ILIOCOSTALIS

Action: Extension and lateral flexion of spine

Origin: 3rd–7th ribs, sacrum, iliac crest, thoracolumbar fascia

Insertion: C4–C6, 1st–6th ribs, 12th rib, thoracolumbar fascia, upper lumbar vertebrae

Agonists: *Extension:* longissimus, spinalis, semispinalis. *Lateral flexion:* longissimus, external/internal oblique (opposite side of lateral flexion)

Poses: *Contracts and lengthens:* parivrtta parsvakonasana (opposite sides), parsva urdhva hastasana

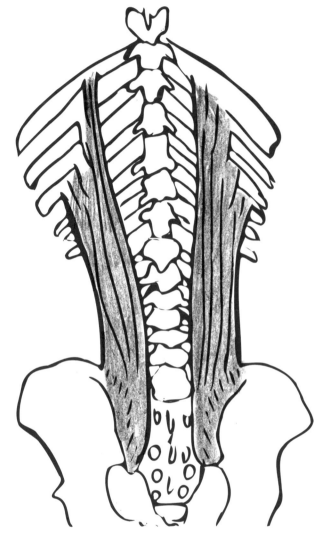

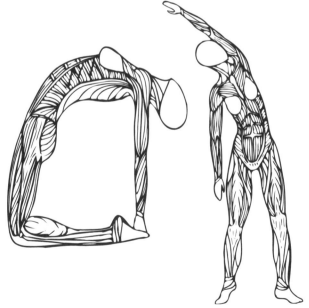

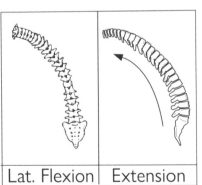

| Lat. Flexion | Extension |

QUADRATUS LUMBORUM

The quadratus lumborum muscle is located on either side of the spine and extends from the hipbones to the ribs. Originating on the iliocolumbar ligaments and iliac crest, the quadratus lumborum fibers extend and insert onto the inferior border of the twelfth ribs and the L1–L4 transverse processes. When the fibers of the quadratus lumborum contract, the spine is brought into lateral flexion. Urdhva hastasana (upward salute side bend pose) brings length to one side of the quadratus lumborum while strengthening the other side.

QUADRATUS LUMBORUM

Action: Lateral flexion of the spine

Origin: Iliolumbar ligaments, iliac crest

Insertion: Inferior border of 12th ribs, L1–L4 transverse processes

Agonists: Iliocostalis lumborum, longissimus thoracis, psoas major, external/internal oblique

Antagonists: (on opposing side) iliocostalis lumborum, longissimus thoracis, psoas major, external/internal oblique

Poses: *Contracts and lengthens:* urdhva hastasana, utthita parsvakonasana

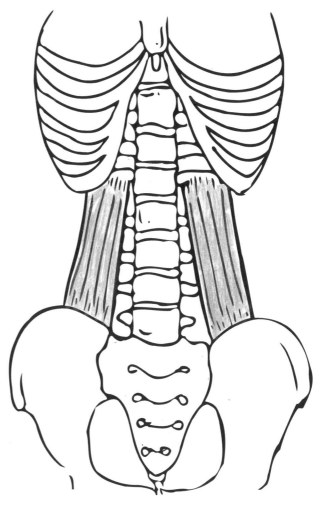

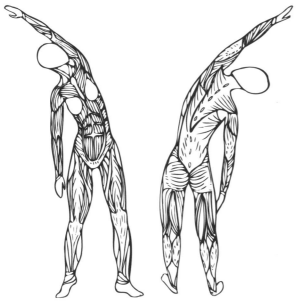

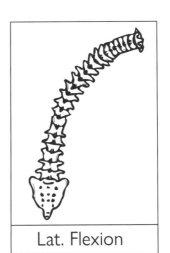

Lat. Flexion

PELVIC BOWL

The bones of the pelvic bowl consist of the two hipbones, the sacrum, and the coccyx. The hipbones start off as three bones: the ilium, the ischium, and the pubis. These bones fuse together as the body grows older to become the hipbones. They then come together to rest against the sacrum to create the sacroiliac joints (SI joints), forming a bowl-shaped structure. The inferior parts of the hipbones include the ischial tuberosities. The ischial tuberosities, known as the "sit bones" in the yoga world, come together to connect the right and left sides of the hips at the pubis symphysis—a cartilaginous joint. Once these pieces come into place, the pelvic bowl is formed. The base of the spine meets with the superior portion of the sacrum and forms the lumbosacral spine, connecting the upper body to the lower body. The head of the femur bone sits in a socket (acetabulum) on the hipbone, forming a ball-and-socket synovial joint called the acetabulofemoral joint. This joint connects the lower body with the upper body. Since the hips are located at the base of the spine, they also support the weight of the spine and upper body during movement. Once the weight is held in the hips, it is transferred into the legs, and then goes into the ground.

Composed of two ball-and-socket joints, the hips are highly mobile and have a wide range of movement. Small and large muscles surround the hip joints to stabilize the pelvic bowl and contract and lengthen to move the femur bone. If a movement muscle group is weak or tight, the hips can become out of balance, which can increase the chances of injury or discomfort.

The movements produced by the hip joints are: adduction, abduction, flexion, extension, internal rotation, and external rotation. To keep the hips in balance, it is important to exercise the hips with a balanced yoga sequence, making sure that the full set of hip movements get lengthening and strengthening exposure.

PELVIC BOWL

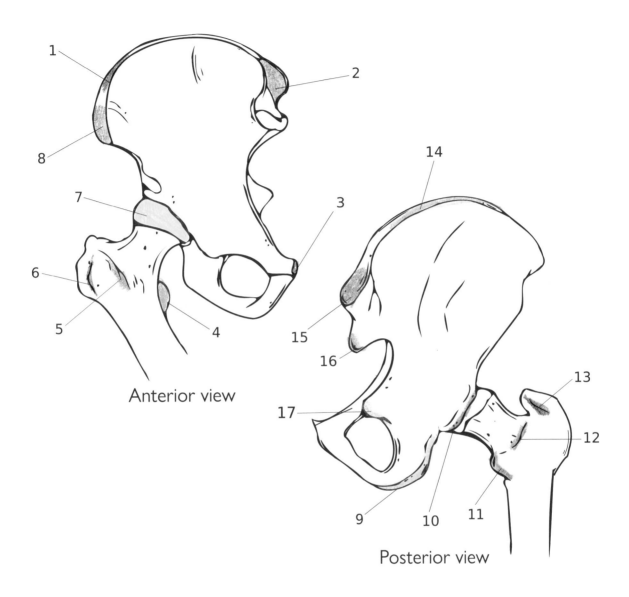

Anterior view

Posterior view

Anterior View
1. Iliac crest
2. Sacroiliac joint site
3. Pubic tubercle
4. Lesser trochanter
5. Intertrochanteric line
6. Greater trochanter
7. Head of femur
8. Anterior superior iliac spine

Posterior View
9. Ischial tuberosity
10. Acetabular rim
11. Lesser trochanter
12. Intertrochanteric crest
13. Greater trochanter
14. Iliac crest
15. Posterior superior iliac spine
16. Posterior inferior iliac spine
17. Ischial spine

PELVIC BOWL

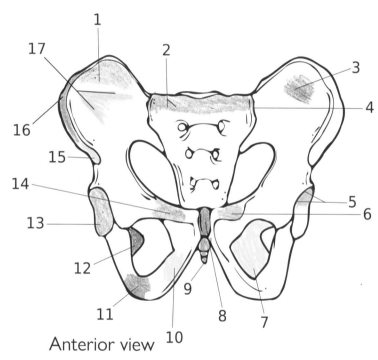

Anterior view

Anterior View
1. Hip bone
2. Sacrum
3. Iliac fossa
4. Sacroiliac joint
5. Acetabular margin
6. Pubic tubercle
7. Obturator foramen
8. Pubic symphysis
9. Coccyx
10. Inferior pubic ramus
11. Ischial ramus
12. Ischial spine
13. Acetabulum
14. Superior pubic ramus
15. Anterior superior iliac spine
16. Iliac crest
17. Gluteal surface

PELVIC BOWL

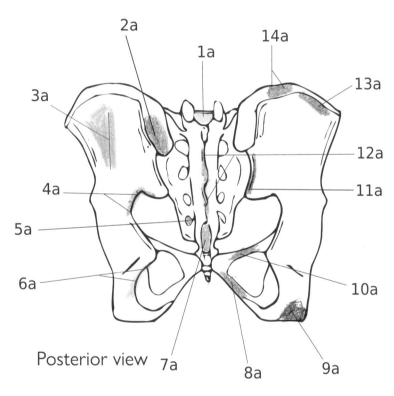

2a
14a
1a
13a
3a
12a
4a
11a
5a
6a
10a
Posterior view
7a
8a
9a

Posterior View
1a. Sacral canal
2a. Posterior superior iliac spine
3a. Iliac wing
4a. Greater sciatic notch
5a. Posterior sacral foramina
6a. Lesser sciatic notch
7a. Sacral hiatus
8a. Inferior pubic ramus
9a. Ischial tuberosity
10a. Superior pubic ramus
11a. Posterior inferior iliac spine
12a. Median sacral crest
13a. Iliac tubercle
14a. Iliac crest

SACRUM

The sacrum is situated between the two hipbones of the pelvis. Triangular in shape, the sacrum's area of connection with the hipbones forms the sacroiliac joints (SI joints). The sacrum is made up of vertebrae (S1–S5) that fuse together as the skeleton ages from childhood to adulthood.

Aligning with the spine, the sacrum receives the upper body weight and transfers it to the hipbones, which then transfer the weight down to the legs. Since the sacroiliac joints have very little room for movement, unbalanced weight put on the sacrum can cause the SI joints to become misaligned. This misalignment is where pain can occur. During yoga, SI pain is commonly seen during twisting poses or poses that open up the pelvis in odd ways (triangle pose). The torque created by the twist can often be too much for the SI joints to handle, causing the joint to slip and the ligaments surrounding the joint to bear more force than they were designed for. In order to prevent this from happening, bring awareness to the amount of pressure generated during twist poses and release the twist a little or allow the sit bones to lift a little off the ground (during sitting twists). This will decrease the amount of torque being created from the twist of the spine and release pressure put on the SI joints.

SACRUM

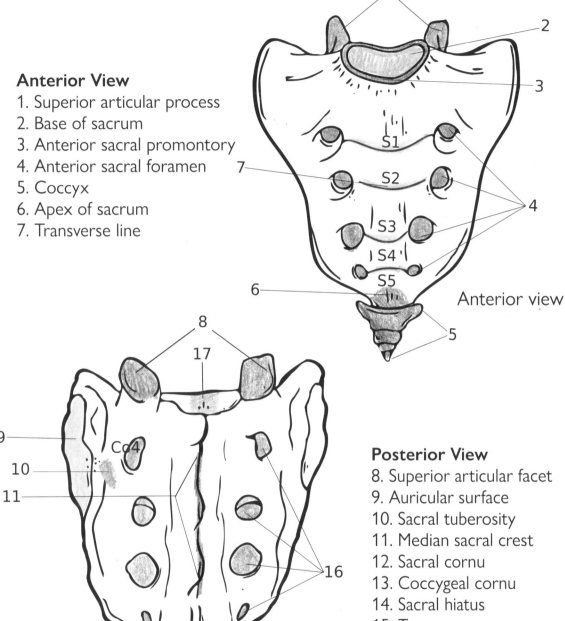

Anterior View
1. Superior articular process
2. Base of sacrum
3. Anterior sacral promontory
4. Anterior sacral foramen
5. Coccyx
6. Apex of sacrum
7. Transverse line

S1
S2
S3
S4
S5

Anterior view

Posterior View
8. Superior articular facet
9. Auricular surface
10. Sacral tuberosity
11. Median sacral crest
12. Sacral cornu
13. Coccygeal cornu
14. Sacral hiatus
15. Transverse process
16. Posterior sacral foramen
17. Sacral canal

Co4
Co1
Co2
Co3

Posterior view

FEMUR BONE AND MUSCLES OF THE HIP

The femur bone is the longest bone in the body and is designed to hold weight. This long bone receives upper body weight from the hips and sends it down to the feet to transfer into the ground. On the proximal end of the bone is the head and neck of the femur. The head is ball-shaped and fits inside the hip socket, creating the acetabulofemoral joint, or the hip joint. The ball-and-socket joint is surrounded in ligaments, cartilage, and synovial fluid. The ligaments work to keep the head and neck of the femur bone situated inside the socket, while the cartilage and synovial fluid lubricate the bone to reduce friction and provide nutrients to the joint. Around the hip joints are small muscles that support and stabilize the head and neck of the femur in the hip socket, in addition to producing internal and external rotation of the femur bone. Larger muscles run the length of the femur bone, contracting to produce larger movements. Along the femur bones are grooves and protuberances. These sites give clues to where muscles and ligaments attach to the bone. As a yoga teacher, it is not necessary to know every groove or protuberance, but getting familiar with them may help bring a deeper understanding of what the muscles look like attached to the femur bone.

FEMUR BONE

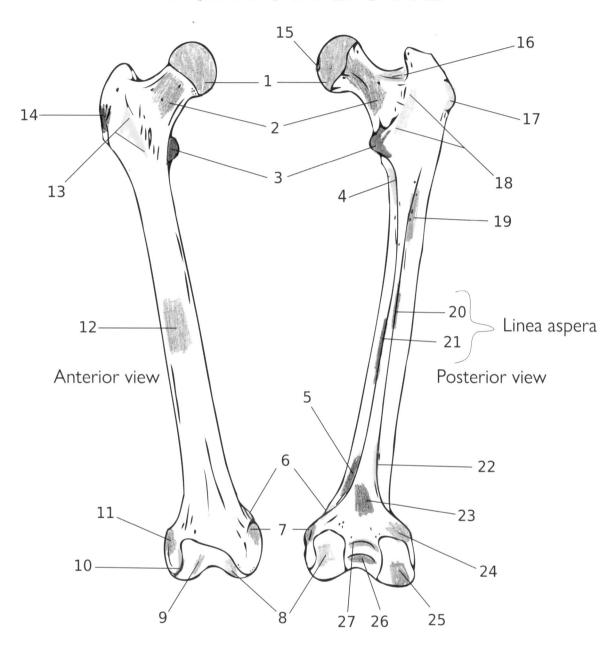

Anterior view

Posterior view

Linea aspera

1. Head
2. Neck
3. Lesser trochanter
4. Pectineal line
5. Medial supracondylar line
6. Medial epicondyle
7. Adductor tubercle
8. Medial condyle
9. Patellar surface

10. Lateral condyle
11. Lateral epicondyle
12. Shaft
13. Intertrochanteric line
14. Greater trochanter
15. Fovea
16. Trochanteric fossa
17. Greater trochanter
18. Intertrochanteris crest

19. Gluteal tuberosity
20. Lateral lip
21. Medial lip
22. Lateral supracondylar line
23. Popliteal surface
24. Lateral epicondyle
25. Lateral condyle
26. Intercondylar notch
27. Intercondylar line

MUSCLES OF THE HIP

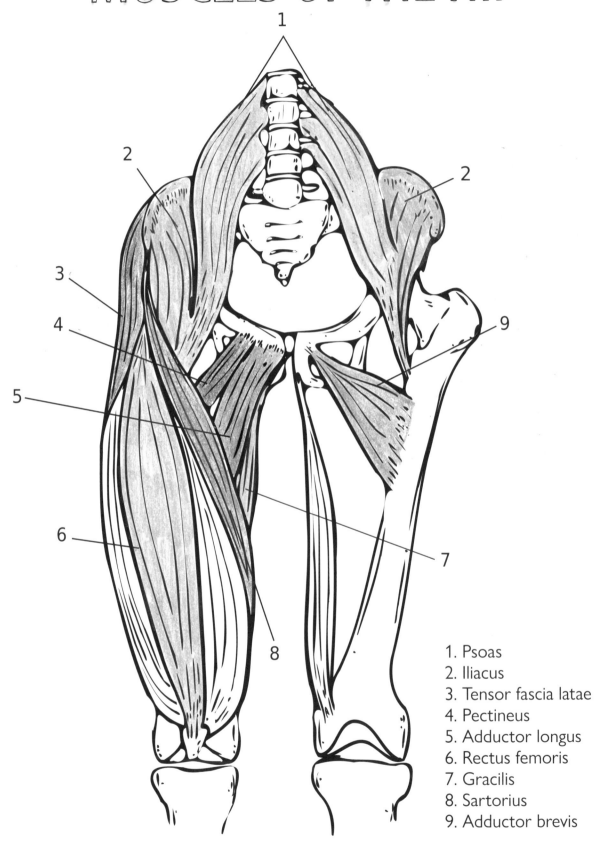

1. Psoas
2. Iliacus
3. Tensor fascia latae
4. Pectineus
5. Adductor longus
6. Rectus femoris
7. Gracilis
8. Sartorius
9. Adductor brevis

MUSCLES OF THE HIP

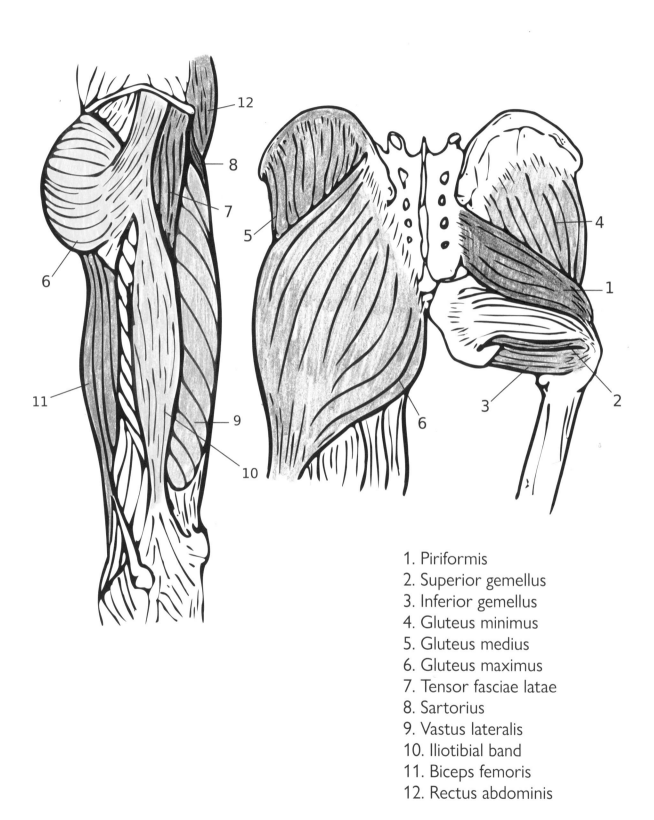

1. Piriformis
2. Superior gemellus
3. Inferior gemellus
4. Gluteus minimus
5. Gluteus medius
6. Gluteus maximus
7. Tensor fasciae latae
8. Sartorius
9. Vastus lateralis
10. Iliotibial band
11. Biceps femoris
12. Rectus abdominis

MUSCLES OF THE HIP

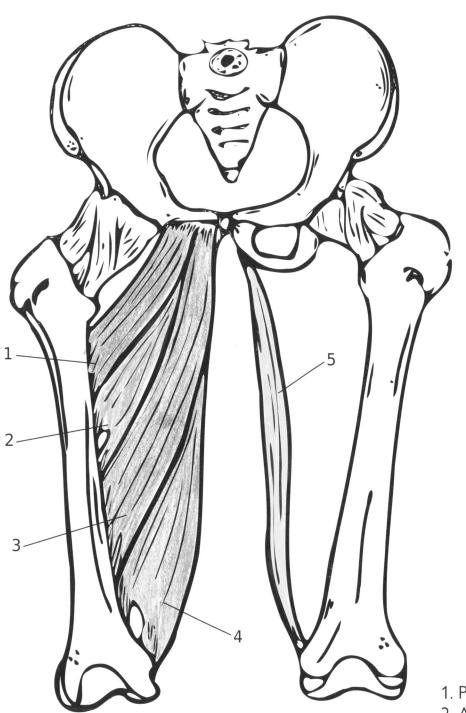

1. Pectineus
2. Adductor brevis
3. Adductor longus
4. Adductor magnus
5. Gracilis

MUSCLES OF THE HIP

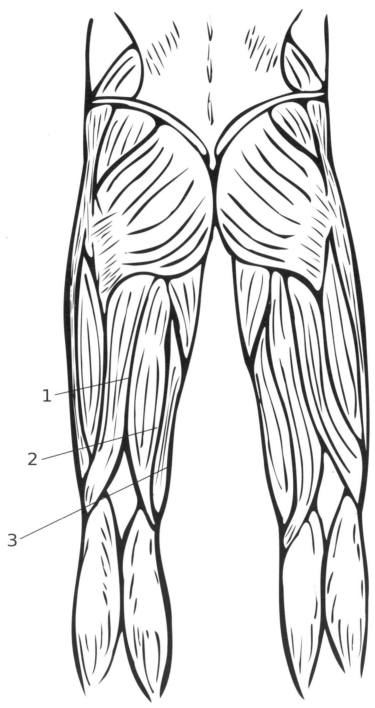

1. Biceps femoris
2. Semitendinosus
3. Semimembranosus

PELVIC FLOOR

The pelvic floor is a sheet of layered muscles that span across the bowl, or opening, of the pelvis. During movement, these muscles contract and lengthen with the body in order to support the pelvic organs and the bottom of the trunk. Coupled with the abdominals, the use of these muscles creates a stronger and more balanced foundation for yoga poses and daily activities. The two muscles that make up the pelvic floor are: the levator ani and the coccygeus. The levator ani can be broken up into three sections: the puborectalis, the pubococcygeus, and the iliococcygeus. Like any muscle, the pelvic floor muscles can become overly active or inactive. In order to bring balance to the pelvic floor, creating an awareness of the state of the muscles is important. Then, decisions about how to relax or strengthen the muscles can be made. A balanced pelvic floor brings a lightness and ease of support to yoga poses and movements and can work to bring the body into a healthier state. Get to know the pelvic floor by learning about the muscles and structures. Color in the areas and familiarize yourself with the names.

PELVIC FLOOR

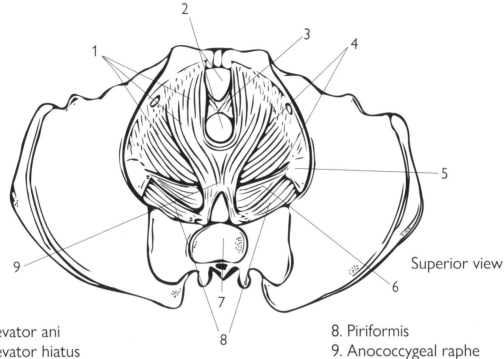

Superior view

1. Levator ani
2. Levator hiatus
3. Prerectal fibers
4. Levator ani tendinous arch
5. Ischial spine
6. Coccygeus
7. Sacrum

8. Piriformis
9. Anococcygeal raphe
10. Pubic symphysis
11. Acetabulum
12. Ischial tuberosity
13. Coccyx
14. Obturator internus

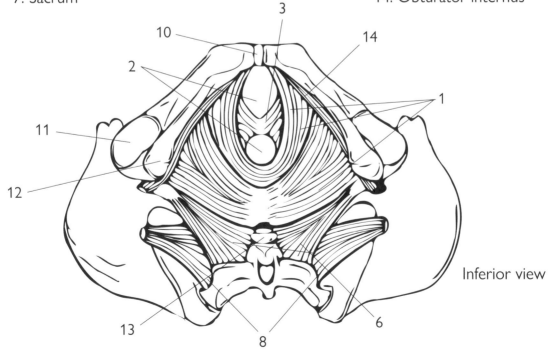

Inferior view

HIP ABDUCTION AND HIP ADDUCTION

The muscles of hip abduction and adduction move the femur bones away from (abduction) and towards (adduction) the midline of the body. The muscles are commonly referred to as "hip abductors" and "hip adductors." These muscles also help the hip joint stabilize during movement. When moving the legs, the abductors and adductors stabilize the pelvis to help produce a more efficient movement. And vice versa: while moving the pelvis with the legs in a fixed position, the abductors and adductors stabilize the femur bone to help produce a more efficient movement.

To activate the hip abductors
To feel the hip abductors contract, begin in mountain pose with your feet hip distance apart. Lift your right foot off the ground slightly, so you are balancing on your left leg. Then, with a slight bend in the left knee, start to bend forwards using the hips. Be sure to keep the spine in a neutral position as you bend forwards, making sure that the bend is coming from the deep flexion of the hips and not the lower back. Straighten back to mountain pose by extending the hips and using the glutes to press your left heel into the floor to stand. Repeat this action 10 times without putting your right foot down onto the floor. Grab a chair or a wall for balance. Switch sides.

What did you notice after repeating this movement? Did the outside muscles of your hip begin to burn? If they didn't, try putting a tight strap above your knees and press out into the strap as you are bending forwards and straightening. This action engages the abductors of the hips and increases pelvic stabilization.

To activate the hip adductors
Grab a yoga block or even a thick book and a chair. Sit in the chair with a neutral spine with your sit bones near the edge of the seat, feet flat on the floor. Place the block in between your thighs, near your knees. Squeeze your legs into the block to hold it in place. Keep the hold for one minute and release. Repeat this action 3–5 times.

What did you notice? Did your inner thighs begin to burn or fatigue?

As you can see, activating the hip abductors and adductors doesn't always require large movements. This is because the muscles engage during small movements as well. Practicing these simple exercises every day will stabilize your pelvis and reduce pain, discomfort, and chance of injury. With a strong pelvis, your balance and mobility will also increase.

HIP ABDUCTION AND HIP ADDUCTION

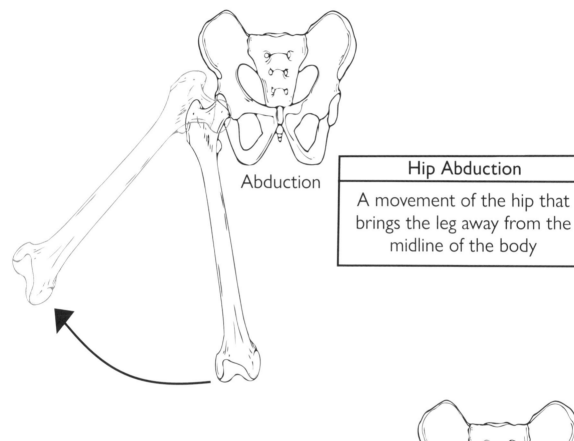

Abduction

Hip Abduction

A movement of the hip that brings the leg away from the midline of the body

Hip Adduction

A movement of the hip that brings the leg in toward or across the midline of the body

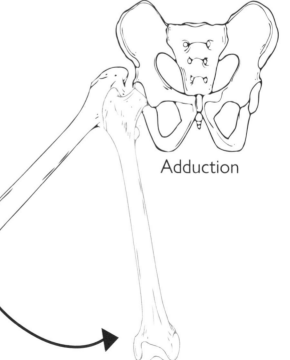

Adduction

HIP ABDUCTORS

Hip abductors are a group of muscles that contract to bring the leg away from the midline of the body. The muscles known as the hip abductors are: the piriformis, the inferior and superior gemellus, the tensor fasciae latae, the gluteus maximus (upper fibers), the sartorius, the gluteus medius, and the gluteus minimus. The hip abductors can become overly tight from prolonged sitting periods and behavioral habits that keep the legs in an abducted position. Over-tightness of a muscle causes the muscle to become shortened, which can eventually cause pain, weakness, and muscle inactivity. Yoga poses or movements that cause the legs to move in towards or across the midline of the body (adduction) can help create length in the abductor muscles. If the abductor muscles become inactive and weak, then yoga poses or movements that require abduction will help strengthen those muscles. The abductors are also responsible for bringing stability to the hip joints during one-legged movements like walking, running, and yoga poses that require one-legged balance. Getting to know the muscles that produce hip abduction can help the mind become aware of the muscles and movements of the hip.

HIP ABDUCTORS

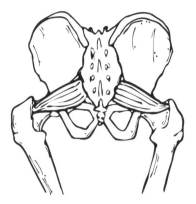

Piriformis

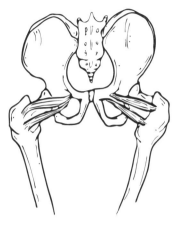

Inferior and superior
gemellus

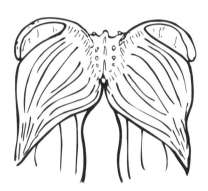

Gluteus maximus
(upper fibers)

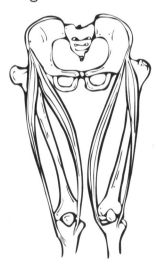

Sartorius with tensor
fasciae latae

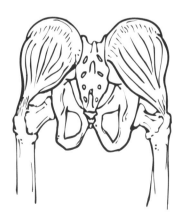

Gluteus medius

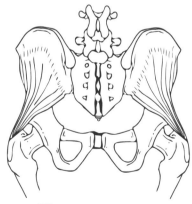

Gluteus minimus

HIP ADDUCTORS

The muscles of hip adduction contract to bring the leg in towards or across the midline of the body. The muscles that produce hip adduction are: the adductor longus, the gracilis, the pectineus, the gluteus maximus (lower fibers), the adductor brevis, and the adductor magnus. Overly tight hip adductors have been known to cause knee, hip, and groin pain. Tight muscles shorten and begin to pull on the sites where the muscles/tendons attach to the bone. In the case of the hip adductors, this is the knee, hip, and groin area. If the muscles are overly tight, gently practice small movements of hip abduction to train the adductors to release and lengthen. Be sure to search for a comfortable feeling of length and to stop movements if pain occurs. If the muscles are weak due to inactivity, the pelvis can become unstable. Participating in movements or yoga poses that require hip adduction can help strengthen those muscles. It is important to have strong and balanced hip adductors (and abductors) because these muscles help create stability of the hips while walking and running.

HIP ADDUCTORS

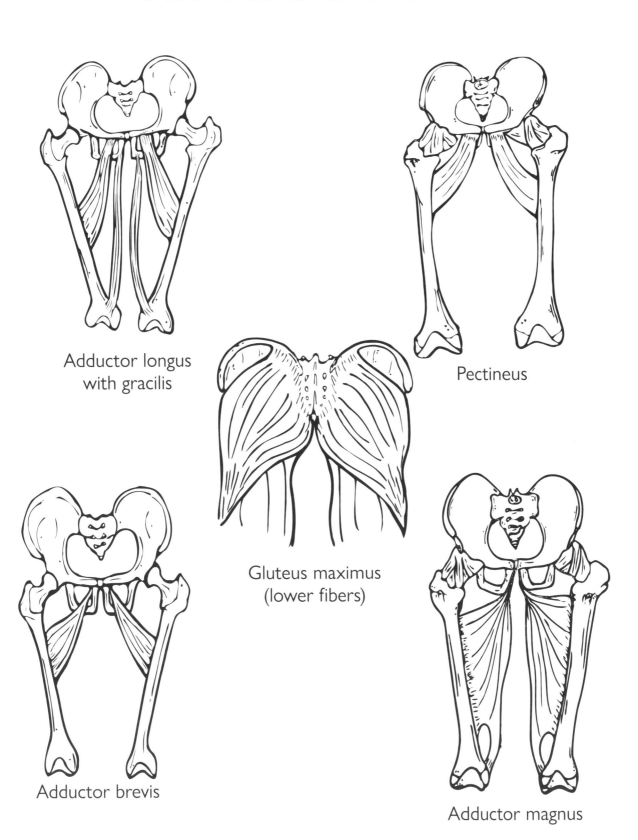

Adductor longus
with gracilis

Pectineus

Gluteus maximus
(lower fibers)

Adductor brevis

Adductor magnus

HIP FLEXION AND HIP EXTENSION

The muscles of hip flexion and extension are also referred as "hip flexors" and "hip extensors." These muscles contract and relax in order to bring the leg forwards (hip flexion) or backwards (hip extension) in space. Hip flexion and extension are the leg movements seen when walking, running, sitting, or standing. These muscles also contract and lengthen to stabilize the pelvis during movement. When practicing hip flexion or extension, stabilizing the pelvis will help the muscles work more efficiently. Since the most common movement of flexion and extension is the act of sitting down and standing up, it is important to learn how to flex and extend at the hips in a safe and efficient way.

To activate the hip extensors
Grab a chair and sit with a neutral spine, sit bones near the edge of the chair, and feet hip distance apart. Align your knees with your ankles and press your feet evenly into the floor. Currently, your hips are in a flexed position.

Before you stand, consciously activate your hip abductors by pressing outwards with your legs (this movement is slight). Lean forwards without bending the spine and prepare to stand. Put your weight into your heels and hover above the chair for a 1–2 seconds. Press the weight down into your heels and extend at the hip until you are standing; give the glutes a little squeeze as you stand back into mountain pose.

What did you notice? How did it feel when consciously putting the weight into your heels to stand? Did you keep your spine in a neutral position or did your lower back bend? Did you feel your glutes engage?

To activate the hip flexors
With the chair behind you, stand in mountain pose with your feet hip distance apart and the chair touching the back of your knees or calves. Without bending in the spine, slowly flex your hips back. Keep your knees aligned over your ankles and engage your abductor muscles by pressing outward with your legs as you flex your hips to lower your pelvis to the chair. Go slow.

What did you notice? Did you feel more pelvic stability as your legs outwardly engaged while flexing your hips to sit down?

Practice sitting in a chair and standing up 10 times. Practicing this daily will increase your conscious awareness of how you sit and stand and will eventually replace a poor postural behaviour with a more improved one.

HIP FLEXION AND HIP EXTENSION

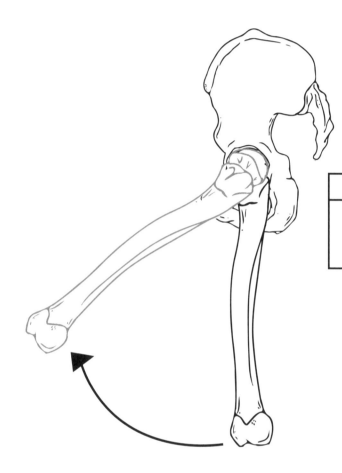

Hip Flexion

A movement that brings the leg forward in space

Hip flexion

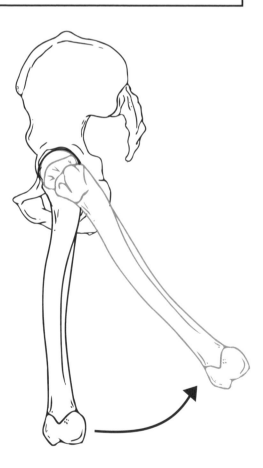

Hip Extension

A movement that brings the leg backward in space

Hip extension

HIP FLEXORS

The hip flexors are a group of muscles that contract to bring the leg forwards in space. The muscles that produce hip flexion are: the iliopsoas, the adductor brevis, the rectus femoris, the sartorius, the tensor fasciae latae, the pectineus, the adductor longus, and the gracilis. Having tight hip flexors is a common issue since the muscles of hip flexion stay contracted during prolonged sitting periods. Tight hip flexors can also mean weak hip flexors. Tight and weak flexion muscles throw off the balance of the hips, leaving other smaller secondary muscles to take on the role of larger primary muscles. This is where pain is seen. For example, the iliopsoas, a muscle consisting of the psoas, psoas minor, and iliacus, is a large muscle that flexes the hips. If the iliopsoas becomes weak, the rectus femoris (a muscle primarily known for flexing the knee and secondarily known for flexing the hips) takes more load than it is designed for. This is why sometimes weak and tight hip flexor pain can be felt near the superior part of the knee. Yoga poses or movements that bring the leg into extension can bring length to the hip flexors. Once the hip flexors become lengthened, yoga poses or movements that require hip flexion can work to strengthen the newly lengthened muscles. This will help balance out the use of the hip flexor muscles and decrease stress on the body caused by misuse. Learning about which muscles produce the hip flexion movement will help increase mind–body awareness of this muscle group in the body. Color in the muscles while imagining how they are working in your body.

HIP FLEXORS

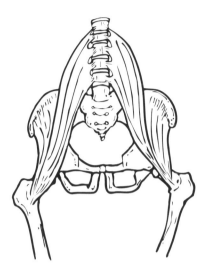

Iliopsoas

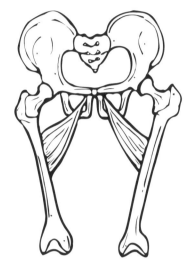

Adductor brevis

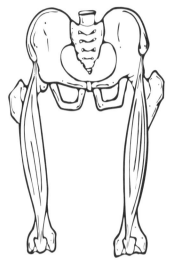

Rectus femoris

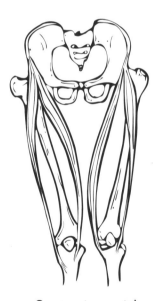

Sartorius with
tensor fasciae latae

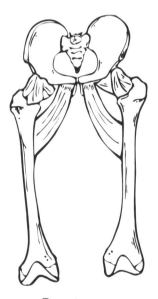

Pectineus

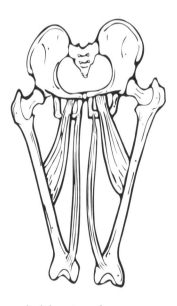

Adductor longus
with gracilis

HIP EXTENSORS

The hip extensors are a group of muscles that contract to extend the thigh backwards in space. If these muscles become overly tight, the ability to flex the hips can be limited. Since overly tight muscles become shortened, students with tight hip extensors may be unable to perform poses that require deep flexion of the hips, that is, child's pose, forwards folds, etc. An inability to contract the hip flexors can lead to weakened hip flexor muscles, causing the muscles of the hips to become unbalanced. To lengthen short hip extensors, yoga poses and movements that bring the legs into slight flexion (depth of flexion will increase over time) will help the muscles lengthen back towards resting length. Conversely, if the hip extensor muscles become weakened from inactivity, an inability to perform yoga poses or movements that require extension can occur. If the body partakes in prolonged periods of sitting, the weight from the body can put pressure on these muscles, causing them to become weak and painful. To strengthen the hip extensors, practice sitting and getting up from a chair. From a sitting position, put your hips feet distance apart and put your weight into your heels. Load your weight into your hips and hoist yourself off the chair. Engage your abductors by slightly pressing your thighs outwards (this will stabilize the hips). From a standing position, load the weight into your heels and begin to fold at the hips by pressing your hips back towards the chair. Keep the lower legs fixed and your knees aligned with your ankles. Press the legs outwards to engage the abductors and to stabilize the pelvis.

HIP EXTENSORS

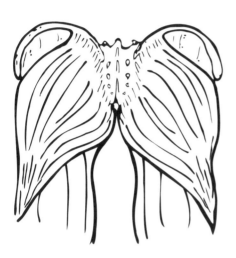

Gluteus maximus

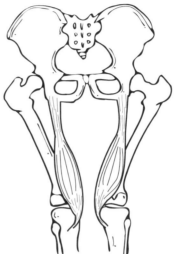

Semimembranosus

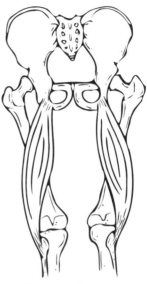

Biceps femoris

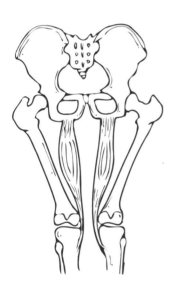

Semitendinosus

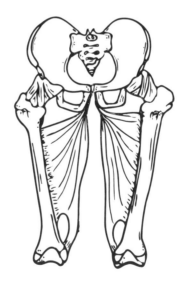

Adductor magnus

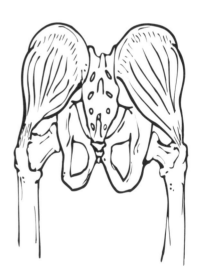

Gluteus medius

EXTERNAL AND INTERNAL HIP ROTATION

External and internal hip rotation are the movements that occur when hip muscles contract and relax to rotate the femur bone away from (external rotation) or towards (internal rotation) the midline of the body. These muscles also help to stabilize and support the pelvis. When practicing these movements, keep the pelvis stable in order to isolate the muscles of the movement. These groups of muscles are also referred to as the "internal rotators" and "external rotators" of the hip.

To activate the external rotators of the hip
Begin sitting in a chair with a neutral spine, sit bones near the edge of the chair with feet hip distance apart. Straighten your right leg out. With the movement originating in your hip joint, turn your femur bone outwards so that your toes point out to the right. Hold this position for 30 seconds.

What did you notice? Did your hip muscles fatigue fast? Did they cramp up or feel weak?

To activate the internal rotators of the hip
Beginning from the same seated position, straighten your right leg out and with the movement originating in your hip joint, turn your femur bone inwards towards the midline of your body so that your toes are pointing left. Hold this position for 30 seconds.

What did notice? Did internal rotation feel easier than external rotation? Did your muscles feel weak or cramp?

Repeat these two movements 3–5 times and then switch legs. Practicing these movements daily will strengthen the hip joint and increase pelvic stabilization.

Note: In order to fully activate the rotators of the hips and to prevent injury from an unbalanced movement of torque, it is important for the origin of the movement to begin within the hip joint and rotate down the leg to the foot, rather than having the movement originate at the ankle and rotate up the leg into the hip.

EXTERNAL AND INTERNAL HIP ROTATION

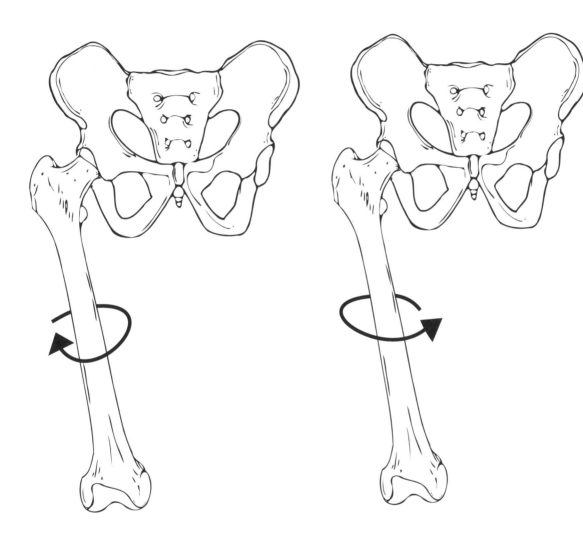

External Rotation
The leg rotates away from the midline of the body

Internal Rotation
The leg rotates toward the midline of the body

HIP EXTERNAL ROTATORS

The external rotators of the hip are a group of muscles that are located on the lateral side of the hip (also referred to as the lateral rotators). When these muscles contract, they rotate the thigh away from the midline. The muscles that make up the hip external rotators are: the piriformis, the obturator externus and obturator internus, the gluteus maximus (lower fibers), the superior gemellus and inferior gemellus, and the quadratus femoris. These muscles are small in size and run across the hip joints deep inside the pelvis. When these muscles are overly active, they can become short from extended contraction and can create pains in the outer hip. Yoga poses or movements with internal rotation of the leg will begin to lengthen out these muscles, bringing them back to resting length. If these muscles become overly inactive, they can become weak and cause imbalances in the pelvis, leading to pain and increased chance of injury. Yoga poses or movements that require external rotation will begin to strengthen these muscles, bringing muscular support and balance back to the hips. Getting to know these muscles as a group will help increase the awareness of these muscles in the hips. As you color in the muscles, keep in mind the function they perform together so it will be engrained in your memory.

HIP EXTERNAL ROTATORS

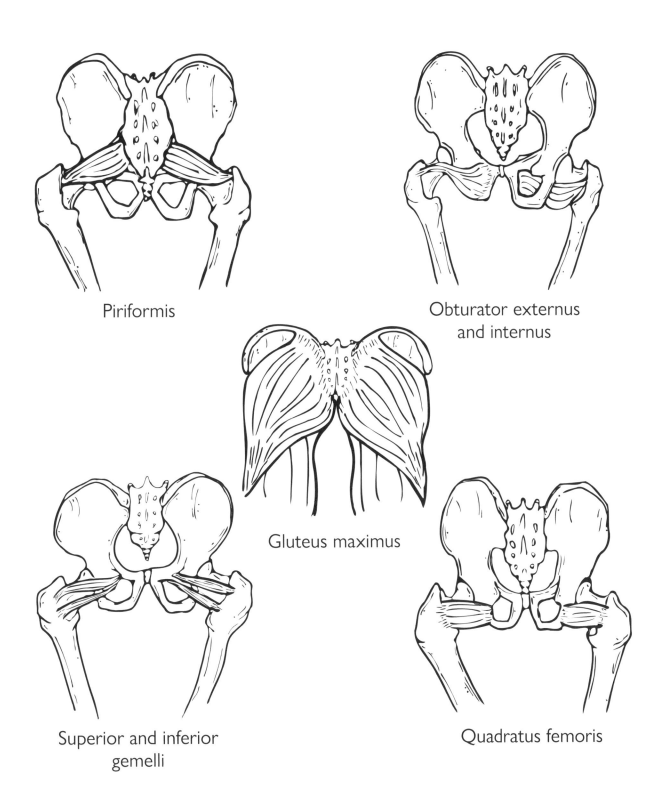

Piriformis

Obturator externus
and internus

Gluteus maximus

Superior and inferior
gemelli

Quadratus femoris

HIP INTERNAL ROTATORS

Hip internal rotation is a movement caused by the contraction of a group of muscles located in the hip, the internal rotators (also referred to as the medial rotators). When these muscles contract, the thigh rotates inward towards the midline of the body. The muscles that create this movement are: the gluteus medius, the adductor longus, the gluteus minimus, the adductor brevis, and the tensor fasciae latae. If these muscles become overly active, the muscles can shorten due to consistent contraction. This can cause pain and imbalances in the hip area. In order to lengthen these muscles, poses or movements that require external rotation of the thigh will begin to bring length to the internal rotators. If these muscles become inactive and weak, the support of the pelvis can become unbalanced and pain or increased chance of injury can arise. Yoga poses or movements that require internal rotation can strengthen these muscles, bringing balance and support to the pelvic area. Learning about the internal rotators can bring awareness to the internal rotation in each pose. With awareness, the mind and body can work together to discover imbalances and figure out ways to bring evenness to the body.

HIP INTERNAL ROTATORS

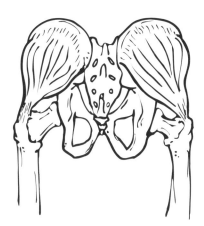

Gluteus medius

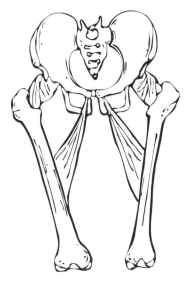

Adductor longus

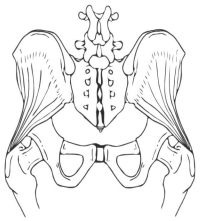

Gluteus minimus

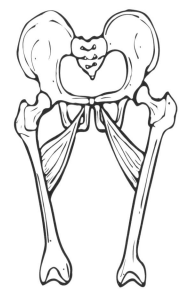

Adductor brevis

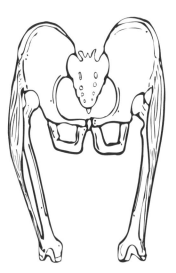

Tensor fasciae latae

ADDUCTOR BREVIS

The adductor brevis originates on the inferior pubic ramus of the pelvis and attaches to the middle third of the linea aspera on the femur bone. The adductor brevis sits deep to the pectineus and adductor longus on the inner thigh. The adductor brevis belongs to the hip adductor group and is the smallest and shortest muscle of the five hip adductors. The primary role of the muscle is to bring the leg in towards the midline. If the inner thigh muscles are tight, yoga poses that bring the leg into abduction will help lengthen the adductors. If the adductors become weak, the pelvis can lose stability, which can affect the balance of the pelvis while in motion. To strengthen the adductors, yoga poses that bring the leg in towards the midline will work to bring strength to the adductors, including the adductor brevis.

ADDUCTOR BREVIS

Action: Adduction and flexion of hip joint (70+ degrees), extension (80+ degrees flexion), pelvic stabilization, internal rotation

Origin: Inferior pubic ramus

Insertion: Middle third of linea aspera on femur

Agonists: *Adduction:* adductor magnus, adductor longus. *Flexion:* iliopsoas, pectineus, tensor fasciae latae

Antagonists: *Adduction:* gluteus maximus, gluteus medius, gluteus minimus. *Internal rotation:* obturator internus, obturator externus, gemellus superior, gemellus inferior, quadratus femoris

Poses: *Contracts:* adho mukha vrksasana, navasana, sirsasana, gomukhasana. *Lengthens:* utkata konasana, prasarita padottanasana, upavista konasana

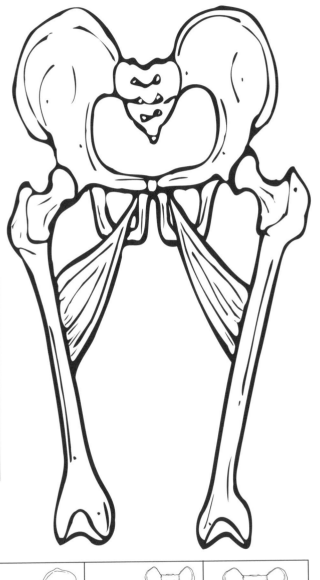

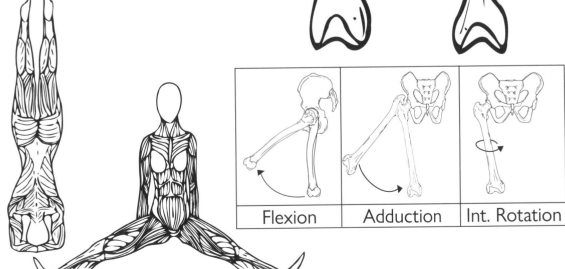

| Flexion | Adduction | Int. Rotation |

ADDUCTOR LONGUS

The adductor longus is part of the hip adductor group. It originates from the anterior superior surface of the pubis and extends down to insert onto the lower two thirds of the linea aspera of the femur bone. When the fibers of the adductor longus contract, the femur bones adduct, internally rotate, and flex at the hip joint. When the adductor longus becomes tight and weak, the ability to strongly bring the legs in towards the midline decreases and the ability to balance in inverted poses may be affected. To lengthen, yoga poses or movements that abduct, externally rotate, and extend the femur bone at the hip joint will begin to elongate the adductor longus. To strengthen the muscles, yoga poses or movements that require adduction, flexion, or internal rotation will work to bring strength to the inner thigh muscles. Salambhasana (locust pose) and sirsasana (headstand pose) are two poses that require adduction of the thighs and will eventually bring strength to the adductor longus.

ADDUCTOR LONGUS

Action: Adduction, internal rotation, and flexion of thigh at hip

Origin: Anterior superior surface of pubis

Insertion: Lower two thirds of linea aspera

Agonists: *Adduction:* adductor magnus, adductor brevis. *Internal rotation:* tensor fasciae latae, gluteus minimus, gluteus medius. *Flexion:* iliopsoas

Antagonists: *Adduction:* gluteus maximus, gluteus medius, gluteus minimus, adductor magnus. *Internal rotation:* obturator internus, obturator externus, gemellus superior, gemellus inferior, quadratus femoris. *Flexion:* gluteus maximus, semitendinosus, semimembranosus, biceps femoris long head, adductor magnus

Poses: *Contracts:* dandasana, navasana, adho mukha vrksasana, sirsasana. *Lengthens:* prasarita padottanasana

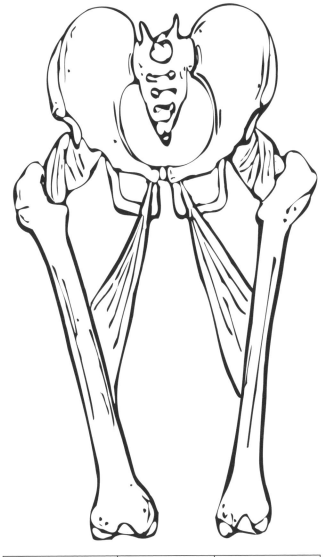

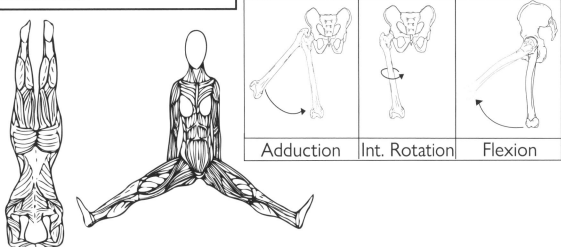

| Adduction | Int. Rotation | Flexion |

ADDUCTOR MAGNUS

The adductor magnus gets its name from its size. It originates on the pubis of the pelvis, travels down the length of the medial thigh, and inserts onto the whole length of the linea aspera of the femur bone. The adductor magnus is a powerful thigh adductor and is the largest muscle of the adductors group. This muscle is unique because of the different angles of fibers in the muscles. The horizontal fibers on the superior part of the muscle contract to assist with flexion of the hip, while the vertical fibers assist with extension of the hip. If the inner thigh muscles become tight, yoga poses that require abduction, flexion, and extension will help release and lengthen the entire muscle.

ADDUCTOR MAGNUS

Action: Adduction of leg at hip, extension of leg at hip, slight flexion, stabilization of pelvis

Origin: Inferior pubic ramus, ischial ramus, ischial tuberosity

Insertion: Medial lip of linea aspera, adductor tubercle of femur

Agonists: *Adduction:* adductor brevis, adductor longus. *Extension:* gluteus maximus, semitendinosus, semimembranosus, biceps femoris long head. *Flexion:* iliopsoas

Antagonists: *Adduction:* gluteus maximus, gluteus medius, gluteus minimus. *Extension:* psoas major, iliacus

Poses: *Contracts:* dandasana, adho mukha vrksasana, gomukhasana, navasana. *Lengthens:* supta baddah konasana, upavistha konasana

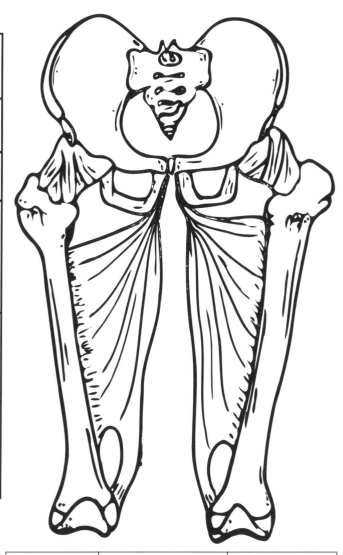

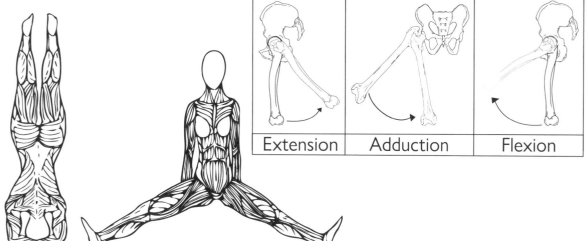

Extension | Adduction | Flexion

BICEPS FEMORIS

The biceps femoris is one of the three muscles that make up the hamstring group. It is a multi-headed muscle located on the posterior thigh. The biceps femoris consists of a short head (SH) and a long head (LH). The short head sits deep to the long head and originates on the lateral lip of the linea aspera on the femur bone. The long head originates on the posterior surface of the ischial tuberosities (sit bones). The short and long heads extend down the length of the femur bone and join together to attach their insertion tendons to the head of the fibula bone. Due to the double originations, when contracted the biceps femoris aids in flexion of the knee joint *and* extension of the leg at the hip joint. A tight biceps femoris can limit the hip joint's ability to extend the knee joint and flex the hip joint. When the muscle becomes too tight and short, when trying to lengthen it, the muscle can pull on the attachment sites, causing a pulling sensation at the back of the knee or near the ischial tuberosities (sit bones). This pain indicates that the muscle is pulling on the tendon–bone attachment sites instead of lengthening at the muscle belly (middle of the muscle). This can cause injury to the muscle and may lead to a tearing of the muscle tendon from the bone.

In order to bring length to the tight biceps femoris, it is important to start off with yoga poses or movements that gently bring the knee into extension or the hip into flexion, making sure that the length is pulling from the middle of the muscle (medial posterior thigh) rather than a pulling sensation at the attachment sites. Once the tight muscle is lengthened or part of a consistent yoga sequence, the muscle can be strengthened to provide more support to the knees and hips. In order to bring strength to the muscle, yoga poses or movements that bring the knee into flexion and the hip into extension will work to bring strength to the biceps femoris.

BICEPS FEMORIS

Action: Flexion of knee joint. Extension of leg at hip. Slight internal rotation when knee is flexed

Origin: Posterior surface of ischial tuberosity (LH), lateral lip of linea aspera on middle third of femur (SH)

Insertion: Head of fibula

Agonists: *Flexion:* semitendinosus, semimembranosus. *Hip extension:* gluteus maximus, semitendinosus, semimembranosus, adductor magnus

Antagonists: *Flexion:* vastus lateralis, vastus medalis, vastus intermedius, rectus femoris. *Hip extension:* iliopsoas

Poses: *Contracts:* utkatasana. *Lengthens:* hanumasana.

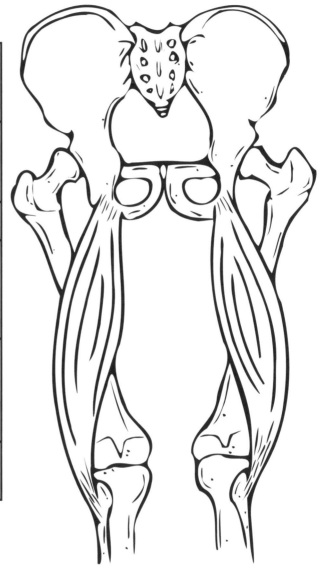

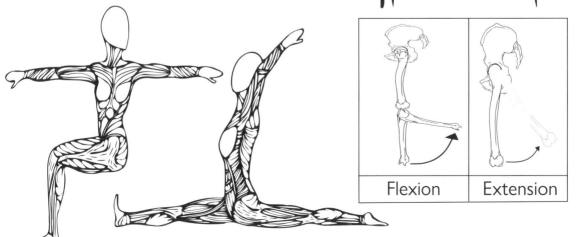

Flexion   Extension

GLUTEUS MAXIMUS

The gluteus maximus is the largest muscle of the "glutes group" (gluteus medius and gluteus minimus) and is the primary muscle for hip extension. The gluteus maximus originates along the sacrum, lumbar fascia, and sacrotuberous ligament. It lies superficially to the gluteus medius and gluteus minimus. Due to the angles of the muscle fibers, the gluteus maximus has two insertion points and can be broken down into two sections: the upper fibers and the lower fibers. The upper fibers assist with abduction of the leg, while the lower fibers assist with adduction of the leg. Together, both the upper and lower fibers work together to extend and externally rotate the leg at the hip joint. The gluteus maximus is known to be one of the strongest muscles in the human body and plays a large role in the stabilization of the hip joint while the body is erect. If the gluteus maximus becomes overly tight, flexion of the hip joint may be limited. If the muscle becomes overly weak, it can result in unstable hips while in motion or standing. Since the hips hold a lot of upper body weight while erect, unstable hips can lead to discomfort and increased chance of injury. To strengthen the gluteus maximus, yoga poses or movements that bring the leg into extension, abduction, and adduction will all work to bring strength and stability to the gluteus maximus and hip area. Going from a seated chair position to standing while putting the weight in the heels and pushing the hips back into flexion is also a good way to strengthen the gluteus maximus.

GLUTEUS MAXIMUS

Action: *Upper fibers:* abduction. *Lower fibers:* adduction. *Entire muscle:* extends and externally rotates leg at hip joint

Origin: Sacrum, ilium, thoracolumbar fascia, sacrotuberous ligament

Insertion: *Upper fibers:* iliotibial tract. *Lower fibers:* gluteal tuberosity

Agonists: *Extension:* semitendinosus, semimembranosus, biceps femoris (LH), adductor magnus. *Abduction:* gluteus medius, gluteus minimus. *External rotation:* obturator internus, obturator externus, gemellus inferior, quadratus femoris

Antagonists: *Extension:* iliopsoas. *Abduction:* adductor longus, adductor brevis, adductor magnus. *External rotation:* tensor fasciae latae, gluteus minimus, gluteus medius

Poses: *Contracts:* salabhasana, ustrasana, urdhva dhanurasana. *Lengthens:* eka pada rajakapotasana (front leg)

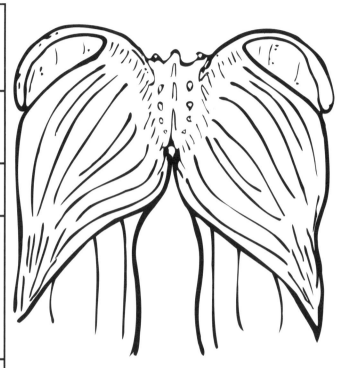

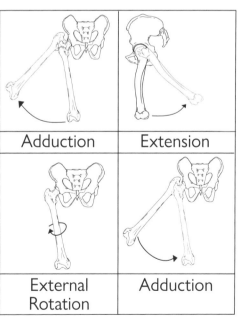

Adduction | Extension

External Rotation | Adduction

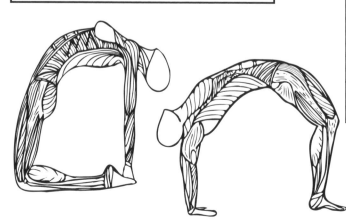

GLUTEUS MEDIUS

The gluteus medius is a muscle located on the posterior side of the hipbones. It lies deep to the gluteus maximus and superficially to the gluteus minimus. The origination of the muscle attaches to the superior posterior part of the hipbone and runs down to cross over the posterior side of the hip joint to attach the insertion tendon to the greater trochanter of the femur bone. Being part of the "glutes group," the gluteus medius works together with the gluteus maximus and minimus to abduct and extend the leg at the hip joint. Due to the angle of the fibers on the muscle of the gluteus medius, the muscle is broken down into two parts: the anterior part and the posterior part. The anterior fibers run at an angle that produces flexion and internal rotation when contracted. The posterior fibers run at an angle that produces extension and external rotation when contracted. The gluteus medius also provides pelvic stabilization when walking, running, or standing. The gluteus medius activates and works to bring balance to the hip area when standing on one leg during poses like vrksasana (tree pose) or ardha chandrasana (half moon pose).

The gluteus medius can become overly tight and weak from prolonged sitting periods. When muscles become overly tight and weak, their ability to perform efficiently decreases and the muscles begin to pull on the attachment sites. When a tight muscle pulls on a bone over a long period of time, it can create imbalances in the skeletal frame. When the gluteus medius becomes tight it is unable to stabilize the pelvis and abduct the thigh efficiently and can also pull on the back of the pelvis. This imbalance can lead to lower back pain or pain that radiates down the leg during weight-bearing exercises like walking or running. Since the gluteus medius performs a number of movements, in order to lengthen the tight muscle, it is important to create a yoga sequence that includes various hip and leg movements. This variety of movement will give the gluteus medius enough range of motion to lengthen and eventually strengthen. It is also important to bring awareness to the gluteus medius while trying to lengthen and strengthen it. Since the muscle may be pulling on the attachment sites, it is imperative to make sure that movement is not causing the gluteus medius to further pull on those attachment sites. This can be felt as a painful pulling sensation in the gluteal region. Search for an angle of movement that brings the stretch to the middle of the muscle. The more you focus on the area, the stronger the mind–body connection with the gluteus medius will become.

GLUTEUS MEDIUS

Action: *Entire muscle:* pelvic stabilization, abduction. *Posterior part:* external rotation and extension of leg at hip. *Anterior part:* flexion, internal rotation

Origin: Ilium

Insertion: Greater trochanter of femur

Agonists: *Abduction:* gluteus maximus, gluteus minimus. *Internal rotation:* tensor fasciae latae, gluteus minimus. *External rotation:* obturator internus, obturator externus, gemellus superior, gemellus inferior, quadratus femoris

Antagonists: *Abduction:* adductor longus, adductor brevis, adductor magnus. *Internal rotation:* obturator internus, obturator externus, gemellus superior, gemellus inferior, quadratus femoris. *External rotation:* tensor fasciae latae, gluteus minimus, gluteus medius

Poses: *Contracts:* salambhasana, salamba bhujangasana. *Lengthens:* gomukhasana

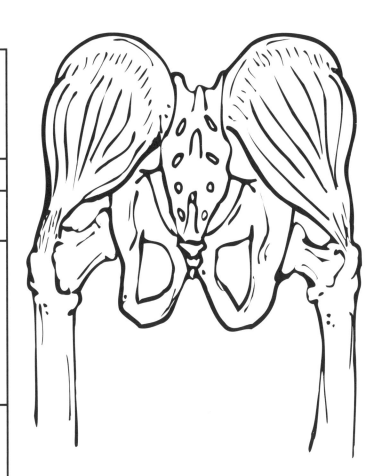

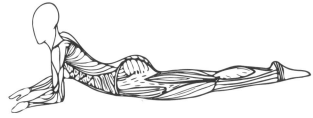

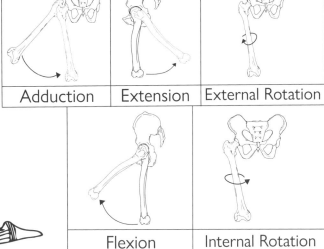

| Adduction | Extension | External Rotation |
| Flexion | Internal Rotation |

GLUTEUS MINIMUS

The gluteus minimus is the smallest of the gluteal muscles and is situated deep to the gluteus medius and the gluteus maximus. It works together with the glutes to produce hip extension and provides stability to the hips. The gluteus minimus originates on the posterior hipbone and runs down to cross the hip joint and attaches to the lateral femur at the greater trochanter. The gluteus minimus can be broken down into two sections: the posterior part and the anterior part. The posterior part contracts to extend and externally rotate the femur bone at the hip joint, while the anterior part contracts to internally rotate and flex the femur bone at the hip joint.

GLUTEUS MINIMUS

Action: *Entire muscle:* abduction, pelvic stabilization. *Anterior:* flexion and internal rotation. *Posterior:* extension and external rotation

Origin: Ilium

Insertion: Greater trochanter of the femur

Agonists: *Abduction:* gluteus maximus, gluteus minimus. *Internal rotation:* tensor fasciae latae

Antagonists: *Abduction:* adductor longus, adductor brevis, adductor magnus. *Internal rotation:* obturator internus, obturator externus, gemellus superior, gemellus inferior, quadratus femoris

Poses: *Contracts:* upavistha konasana, utkata konasana. *Lengthens:* gomukhasana

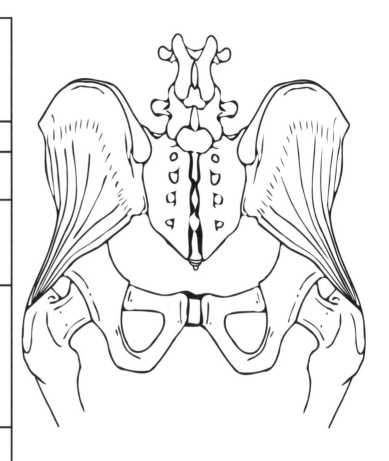

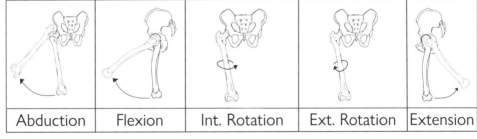

| Abduction | Flexion | Int. Rotation | Ext. Rotation | Extension |

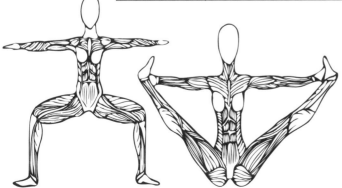

GRACILIS

The gracilis muscle is located on the medial side of the thigh and is the most superficial muscle of the inner thigh compartment. It originates from the inferior pubis ramus and extends down the length of the medial thigh to cross over the knee joint. The insertion tendon joins with the sartorius and semitendinosus tendons to attach to the medial side of the tibial tuberosity. The gracilis is responsible for assisting the hip joint with hip adduction and flexion as well as assisting the knee joint with knee flexion and internal rotation. To lengthen a tight gracilis, bring the body into yoga poses or movements that abduct and extend the hip joint or extend the knee joint.

GRACILIS

Action: Internally rotates leg at hip; adducts leg at hip

Origin: Inferior pubic ramus

Insertion: Medial surface of tibial shaft

Agonists: Iliopsoas, pectineus, sartorius, tensor fasciae latae, adductor brevis

Antagonists: Adductor magnus, gluteus maximus

Poses: *Contracts:* adho mukha vrksasana, garudasana, adho mukha svanasana. *Lengthens:* prasarita padottanasana

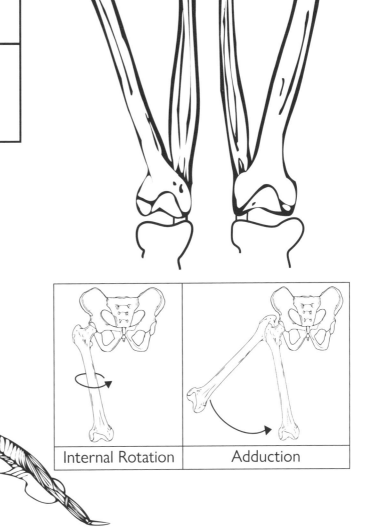

Internal Rotation

Adduction

GEMELLI

The gemelli are made up of two muscles: the inferior gemellus and the superior gemellus. These tiny muscles originate on the ischial spine located on the posterior superior portion of the ischial tuberosities (sit bones). They extend laterally and cross over the posterior hip joint and join with the tendon of the obturator internus, which then inserts onto the medial surface of the greater trochanter. Together, these two muscles are part of the six deep muscles that externally rotate the femur bone. Due to their deep position and proximity to the hip joints, they also work to bring stabilization to the hip joint.

These muscles can become weak and tight from prolonged sitting periods or postural behaviors that keep the thighs externally rotated. This tightness can be felt as pain in the posterior hip joint. To lengthen the gemelli, yoga poses or movements that internally rotate the thigh will elongate the gemelli muscles. To strengthen, yoga poses or movements that externally rotate the legs will work to bring strength to the muscles of external rotation.

GEMELLI

Action: External rotation, adduction, and extension of the hip joint. Abduction of the flexed thigh, hip joint stabilization

Origin: Ischial spine (gemellus superior). Ischial tuberosity (gemellus inferior)

Insertion: Obturator internus tendon (medial surface of greater trochanter)

Agonists: *External rotation:* piriformis, obturator internus, obturator externus, quadratus femoris

Antagonists: *Eternal rotation:* gluteus medius, gluteus minimus (gemellus superior). Iliotibial band, tensor fasciae latae (gemellus inferior)

Poses: *Contracts:* trikonasana baddah konasana, padmasana. *Lengthens:* uttanasana, dandasana

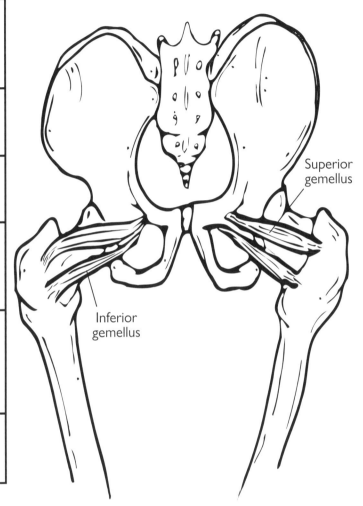

Superior gemellus

Inferior gemellus

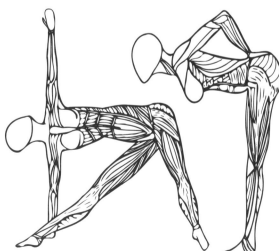

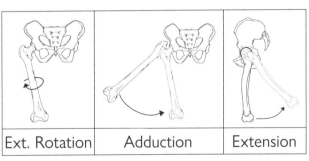

| Ext. Rotation | Adduction | Extension |

ILIOPSOAS

The iliopsoas is made up of three muscles: the iliacus, the psoas major, and the psoas minor. The muscles are grouped together due to the common insertion point between the iliacus and the psoas major. The psoas major originates on the lumbar spine. It attaches to T12–L5 transverse processes of the vertebrae. The psoas minor originates on the lateral surfaces of T12–L1 vertebrae. The iliacus originates on the iliac fossa, which is near the inner lip of the pelvic bowl. The muscles weave together and cross over the anterior part of the hip joint to insert onto the lesser trochanter of the femur bone. The iliopsoas contracts to flex the hips and is the strongest muscle in the hip flexor group. When the iliopsoas becomes tight and weak from prolonged periods of sitting and disuse, assisting hip flexor muscles are recruited to pick up the force required to flex the hips. This can put stress on the rectus femoris of the quadriceps muscles. Since the rectus femoris is designed to assist the iliopsoas in hip flexion, picking up the slack of the iliopsoas puts too much stress on the rectus femoris. This can be felt as pain on the anterior distal portion of the femur bone. A tight iliopsoas can also pull on the origin attachment sites of the lumbar spine, which can put stress on the low back and bring the spine out of alignment. Bringing length and strength to the muscles of the iliopsoas will help the muscle function more efficiently.

To lengthen the iliopsoas, yoga poses and movements that bring the hip into extension will elongate the iliopsoas muscles. Poses like bhujangasana (cobra pose) and the back leg of virabhadrasana I (warrior I) work to lengthen the iliopsoas muscle. Once the muscle has lengthened, working to bring strength to the muscle will increase the amount of force it can produce. To strengthen the iliopsoas muscles, yoga poses and movements that bring the hips into flexion will begin to strengthen the muscles. Adho mukha svanasana (downward facing dog) and navasana (boat pose) bring the hips into flexion and will encourage the iliopsoas to strengthen. It is also important to bring awareness to the area of the muscle while trying to increase length and strength. Getting to know how the muscle feels when being used will increase the mind–body communication with the iliopsoas and can increase the voluntary control over the muscle.

The iliopsoas is important not only for flexion, but also for overall balance of the body while erect. Since it attaches to the lumbar spine and weaves across the hip joint to attach to the femur bone, it is a main muscle that connects the upper body to the lower body. During erect movements it works to laterally stabilize the spine. It is one of the most important muscles for voluntary control over the body and should not be overlooked.

ILIOPSOAS

Action: Flexion and external rotation of hip joint. Lateral flexion. Upward rotation of pelvis (psoas minor)

Origin: T12–L1 lateral surfaces, L1–L5 vertebral surfaces. Iliac fossa (iliacus)

Insertion: Lesser trochanter (psoas major and iliacus). Iliopectineal arch (psoas minor)

Agonists: *Flexion:* psoas major, iliacus, psoas minor, rectus femoris, sartorius

Antagonists: *Flexion:* gluteus maximus, semitendinosus, semimembranosus, biceps femoris, adductor magnus

Poses: *Contracts:* navasana, utkatasana, uttanasana. *Lengthens:* dhanurasana, setu bandha sarvangasana, ustrasana

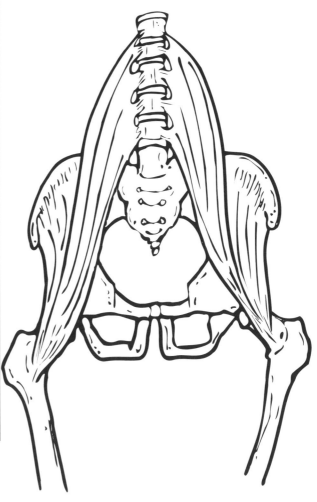

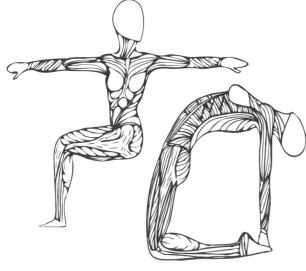

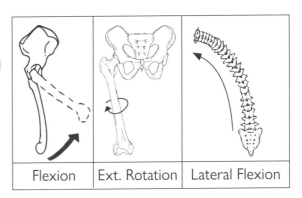

| Flexion | Ext. Rotation | Lateral Flexion |

OBTURATOR EXTERNUS AND INTERNUS

The obturator externus and the obturator internus are two of the six deep muscles that externally rotate the hip joint. They originate on the medial surface of the pubis and run across the hip joint to join tendons with the gemelli. They insert onto the greater trochanter of the femur. Due to the close proximity to the hip joint, the obturator externus and the obturator internus work to stabilize the hip joint as well as work to assist with bringing the hip into adduction and abduction. Tight external rotators can bring weakness to the hip joint and can limit the body's ability to do yoga poses that require a strong external rotation of the hip joint. Practicing ardha chandrasana (half moon pose) can help bring strength to the external rotators of the standing leg.

OBTURATOR EXTERNUS AND INTERNUS

Action: External rotation, adduction, and extension of the hip joint (internus). Abduction of the thigh when the hip is flexed

Origin: Medial surface of pubis

Insertion: Greater trochanter (internus)

Agonists: Piriformis, gemelli, quadratus femoris

Antagonists: Gluteus minimus

Poses: *Contracts:* supta baddah konasana, trikonasana padmasana. *Lengthens:* uttanasana, dandasana

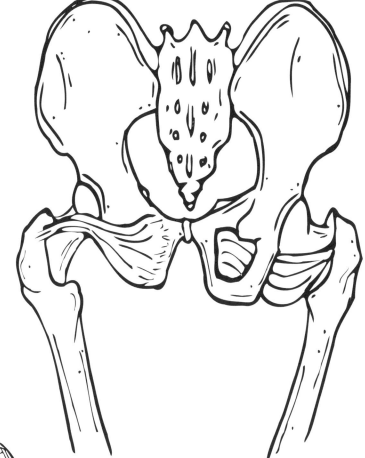

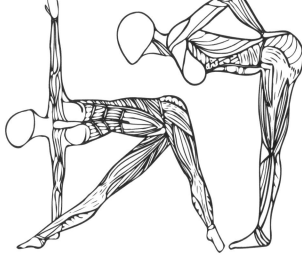

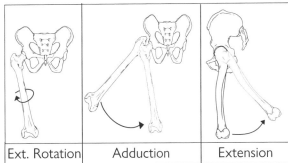

| Ext. Rotation | Adduction | Extension |

PECTINEUS

The pectineus is a small muscle located in the inner compartment of the thigh. Originating from the pubis and inserting onto the pectineal line of the femur, the pectineus contracts to adduct the thighs in towards the midline of the body. The pectineus also assists in flexion and internal rotation of the leg at the hip joint. Poses like bakasana (crow pose), adho mukha vrksasana (handstand), and garudasana (eagle pose) all require the adductors to squeeze in towards the midline of the body. If the adductors of the thighs become too tight, poses like supta baddah konasana (reclined bound angle pose) or movements that require abduction of the thighs will be limited in how far away from the midline the thighs can abduct. To lengthen tight thigh adductors, yoga poses or movements that require slight abduction will help to elongate the pectineus muscles.

PECTINEUS

Action: Adduction, flexion, and internal rotation. Pelvic stabilization

Origin: Pecten pubis

Insertion: Pectineal line of femur

Agonists: *Adduction:* adductor longus, adductor brevis, adductor magnus. *Flexion:* iliopsoas

Antagonists: *Adduction:* gluteus maximus, gluteus medius, gluteus minimus. *Flexion:* gluteus maximus, semitendinosus, semimembranosus, biceps femoris, adductor magnus

Poses: *Contracts:* adho mukha vrksasana, urdhva dhanurasana. *Lengthens:* prasarita padottanasana

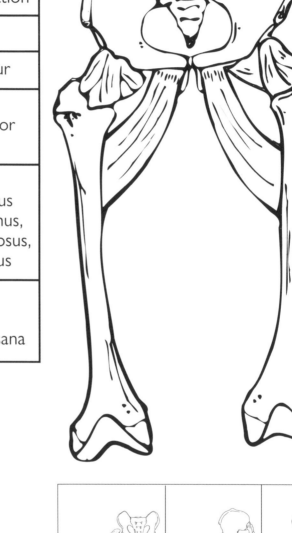

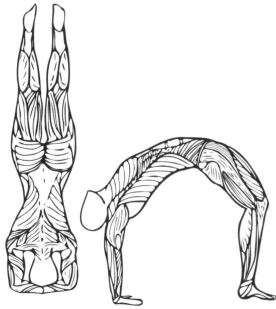

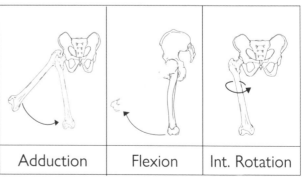

| Adduction | Flexion | Int. Rotation |

PIRIFORMIS

The piriformis is a small muscle that makes up one of the six deep muscles that externally rotate the thigh. It originates on the lateral sides of the inferior sacrum and runs across the superior portion of the hip joint. It joins with the tendon of the obturators and gemelli to insert onto the greater trochanter of the femur. When contracted, the piriformis is responsible for externally rotating and adducting the hip joint. The piriformis also works to stabilize the sacrum during movement. Due to its close proximity to the sciatic nerve, if the piriformis becomes overly tight it can pinch the sciatic nerve. This can cause a dull pain in the hips that runs down the legs to the feet. To bring length to the piriformis, yoga poses or movements that bring the leg into internal rotation or abduction will begin to elongate the piriformis muscle.

PIRIFORMIS

Action: External rotation, abduction, extension of the hip joint, stabilizes pelvis

Origin: Pelvis surface of sacrum

Insertion: Greater trochanter of femur

Agonists: *External rotation:* obturator internus, obturator externus, gemelli, quadratus femoris. *Abduction:* gluteus maximus, gluteus medius, gluteus minimus

Antagonists: *External rotation:* tensor fasciae latae, gluteus minimus, gluteus medius. *Abduction:* adductor longus, adductor brevis, adductor magnus

Poses: *Contracts:* vrksasana, utkata konasana. *Lengthens:* adho mukha svanasana

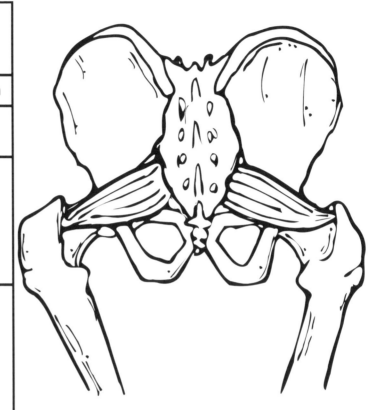

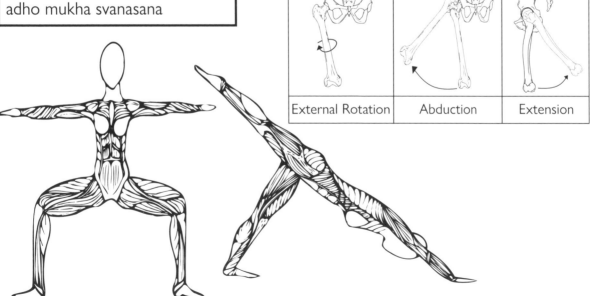

| External Rotation | Abduction | Extension |

QUADRATUS FEMORIS

The quadratus femoris is one of the six deep muscles that are responsible for externally rotating the leg at the hip joint. It is a square muscle that originates on the lateral ischial tuberosity, runs across the posterior portion of the hip joint, and inserts onto the intertrochanteric crest of the femur. In addition to external rotation, the quadratus femoris is responsible for assisting the hip joint in adduction of the leg. The quadratus femoris can become tight from prolonged periods of external rotation due to postural habits. To lengthen the external rotators, yoga poses and movements that bring the leg into internal rotation will begin to elongate the quadratus femoris.

QUADRATUS FEMORIS

Action: External rotation and adduction of hip joint. Abduction of thigh when flexed

Origin: Lateral ischial tuberosity

Insertion: Intertrochanteric crest of the femur

Agonists: Piriformis, gemelli, obturator internus, quadratus femoris

Antagonists: *External rotation:* adductor longus, adductor brevis, gluteus minimus, gluteus medius, tensor fasciae latae, semimembranosus, semitendinosus

Poses: *Contracts:* supta baddah konasana, ananda balasana, utkata konasana. *Lengthens:* dandasana, uttanasana

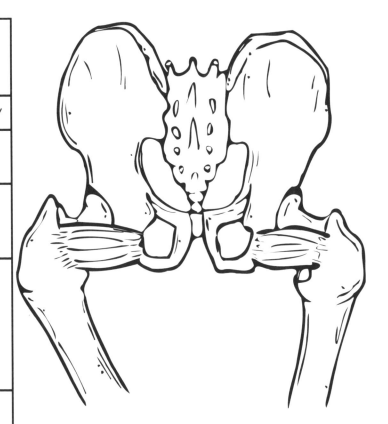

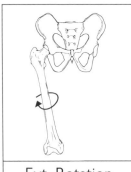

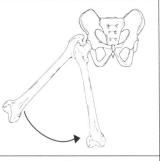

| Ext. Rotation | Adduction |

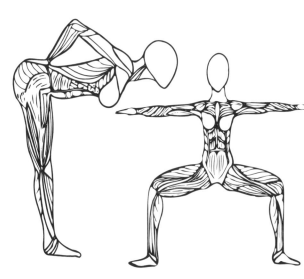

RECTUS FEMORIS

The rectus femoris is one of the four muscles that make up the quadriceps group. Originating from the anterior inferior iliac spine on the pelvis, it crosses over the hip joint and extends down the length of the thighbone. It then crosses over the knee joint and inserts onto the tibial tuberosity of the tibia bone. The rectus femoris works together with the other three muscles that make up the quadriceps (vastus lateralis, vastus medialis, and vastus intermedius) to extend the knee joint. Unlike its common knee extensors, the rectus femoris is also responsible for assisting the iliopsoas in hip flexion. Since the muscle crosses over two joints and is responsible for two large movements, a tight rectus femoris can cause pain at the knee joint and the hip joint. The tight muscle shortens and can begin to pull on the attachment sites. This can increase discomfort and decrease mobility during yoga poses or movements that bring the knee into flexion or the hip into extension. A weak iliopsoas can also put undue stress onto the rectus femoris and can cause pain at the knee joint. In order to lengthen the rectus femoris, yoga poses that bring the knee into slight flexion or the hip into slight extension can begin to lengthen the rectus femoris. A good pose for lengthening is ustrasana (camel pose), which requires both knee flexion and hip extension. Keep in mind that ustrasana is a deep pose and it is good practice to warm the joints up with a well-rounded yoga flow before entering deep poses. When working to bring length to the rectus femoris, if there is any pain at the knee or hip joints, refrain from the yoga pose or movement and figure out a more subtle movement that will bring the stretch to the middle of the muscle.

RECTUS FEMORIS

Action: Flexion of the hip joint, extension of the knee joint

Origin: Anterior inferior iliac spine of the pelvis and acetabular roof of the hip joint

Insertion: Tibial tuberosity

Agonists: *Flexion:* iliopsoas. *Extension:* vastus intermedius, vastus lateralis, vastus medialis

Antagonists: *Flexion:* gluteus maximus, semitendinosus, semimembranosus, biceps femoris, adductor magnus. *Extension:* biceps femoris, semitendinosus, semimembranosus

Poses: *Contracts:* uttanasana, adho mukha svanasana. *Lengthens:* ustrasana, urdhva dhanurasana

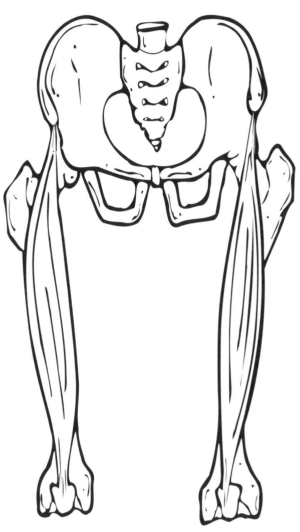

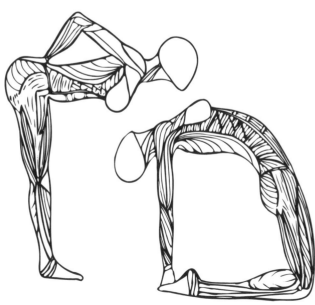

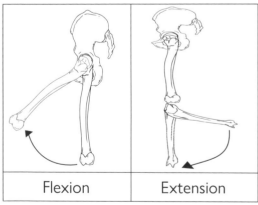

Flexion   Extension

SEMIMEMBRANOSUS

The semimembranosus is one of the three muscles that make up the hamstrings group located on the posterior thigh. Originating on the posterior lateral surface of the ischial tuberosity (sit bone), the semimembranosus extends down the length of the thighbone and crosses over the knee joint to attach to the superior medial condyle of the tibia. When contracted, the semimembranosus shortens to flex the knee joint. The hamstrings are often a high area of focus in yoga due to the amount of flexion the knee sees daily. Bringing too much length to the semimembranosus can cause the attachment to tear at the origination site at the sit bones. It is important to pay attention to the sensations produced when lengthening the hamstrings. A pulling sensation near the sit bones indicates that the hamstrings are being over-stretched and need a break. To prevent over-lengthening of the semimembranosus, make sure that the sensation of stretch is in the middle of the muscle and does not feel painful.

SEMIMEMBRANOSUS

Action: Extension of leg at hip, flexion of knee joint, internal rotation of knee when flexed, pelvic stabilization

Origin: Posterior lateral surface of ischial tuberosity and sacrotuberous ligament

Insertion: Superior medial condyle of tibia, popliteal ligament

Agonists: *Extension:* gluteus maximus, semitendinosus, biceps femoris (LH), adductor magnus. *Flexion:* biceps femoris, semitendinosus. *Internal rotation:* semitendinosus, popliteus

Antagonists: *Extension:* psoas major, iliacus. *Flexion:* vastus lateralis, vastus medialis, vastus intermedius, rectus femoris. *Internal rotation:* biceps femoris

Poses: *Contracts:* virabhadrasana III, dhanurasana, salabhasana. *Lengthens:* hanumasana, utthita trikonasana

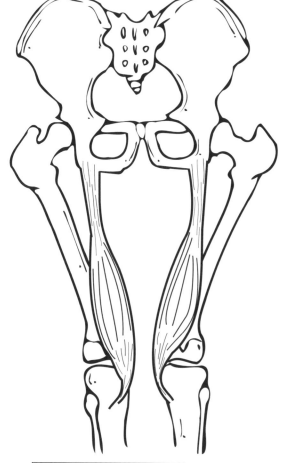

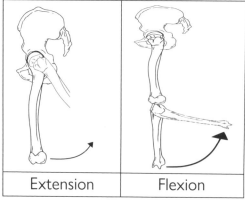

| Extension | Flexion |

SEMITENDINOSUS

The semitendinosus is one of three muscles that make up the hamstrings group. It is the most medial of the muscles and originates on the posterior surface of the ischial tuberosities (sit bones) of the pelvis. The semitendinosus runs down the posterior thigh and crosses over the knee joint to join tendons with the gracilis and sartorius and inserts onto the medial tibial condyle of the tibia bone. Similar to its common knee flexors, the semitendinosus is often in danger of being over-stretched, causing tears of the tendon at the attachment sites. To prevent tearing the tendon, be aware of the sensations in the posterior thigh and make sure the stretch is in the middle of the muscle.

SEMITENDINOSUS

Action: Extension of the leg at hip, flexion of knee joint, internal rotation of knee when flexed

Origin: Posterior surface of ischial tuberosity

Insertion: Medial tibial condyle, popliteal ligament with fibers inserting into popliteal fascia

Agonists: *Extension:* gluteus maximus, semitendinosus, biceps femoris (LH), adductor magnus. *Flexion:* biceps femoris, semitendinosus. *Internal rotation:* semitendinosus, popliteus

Antagonists: *Extension:* psoas major, iliacus. *Flexion:* vastus lateralis, vastus medialis, vastus intermedius, rectus femoris. *Internal rotation:* biceps femoris

Poses: *Contracts:* shalambasana, utkatasana, dhanurasana. *Lengthens:* hanumasana, prasarita padottanasana, utthita trikonasana, ado mukha svanasana

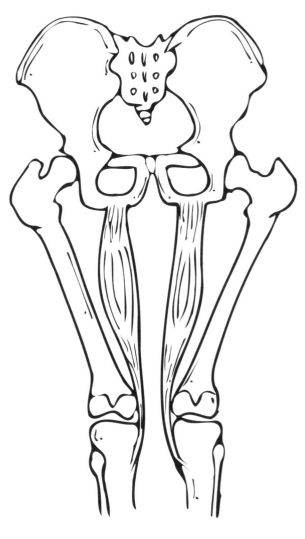

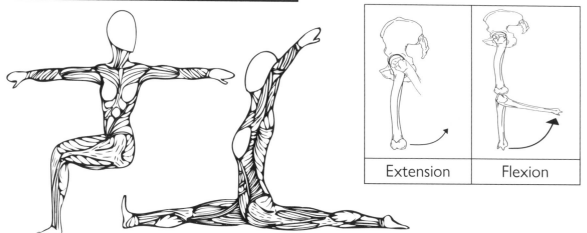

| Extension | Flexion |

TENSOR FASCIAE LATAE

The tensor fasciae latae (TFL) is located on the lateral hip. It originates on the anterior superior iliac spine of the pelvis. It runs down the lateral thigh and inserts into the iliotibial tract (IT band) along with the tendon of the gluteus maximus. The IT band continues down the lateral thigh to attach to the lateral knee and is responsible for stabilizing the knee joint. The contraction of the TFL produces abduction, flexion, and internal rotation of the leg at the hip joint. The TFL can be felt strongly during navasana (boat pose), where the TFL assists in flexion of the hip and internal rotation of the leg at the hip joint. Tightness of the TFL can be felt as a pulling sensation or discomfort in the lateral knee, since the tight TFL shortens and pulls on the attachment of the IT band. To lengthen the TFL, poses that externally rotate, extend, and adduct the hip can bring length to the muscle. Bhujangasana (cobra pose) can work to bring length to the TFL because it extends the hips and adducts the thighs inward towards the midline.

TENSOR FASCIAE LATAE

Action: Tenses the fascia lata, abducts, flexes and internally rotates leg at hip

Origin: Anterior superior iliac spine

Insertion: Iliotibial tract

Agonists: *Internal rotation:* gluteus minimus, gluteus medius. *Abduction:* gluteus maximus, gluteus medius, gluteus minimus. *Extension:* vastus lateralis, vastus medialis, vastus intermedius, rectus femoris. *Flexion:* iliopsoas

Antagonists: *Internal rotation:* gemellus superior/inferior, obturator internus/externus, quadratus femoris. *Abduction:* adductor longus, adductor brevis, adductor magnus. *Extension:* biceps femoris, semitendinosus, semimembranosus. *Flexion:* gluteus maximus, semitendinosus, semimembranosus, biceps femoris, adductor magnus

Poses: *Contracts:* utkatasana konasana, supta baddah konasana. *Lengthens:* bhujangasana, supta virasana

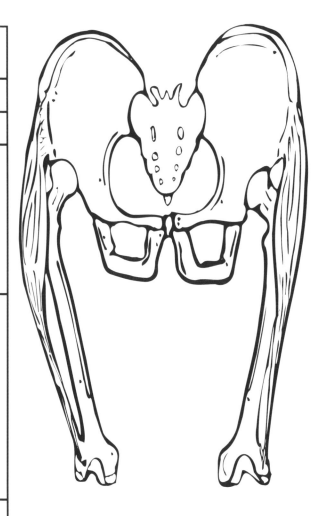

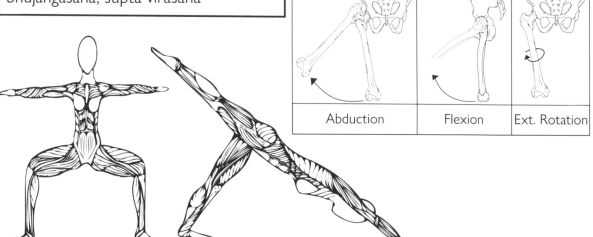

| Abduction | Flexion | Ext. Rotation |

THE KNEES

The knee joint is a complex hinge joint and is formed by articulations between three bones: the femur, the tibia, and the patella. Ligaments, tendons, muscles, and nerves surround the knee joint and contribute to stabilizing and moving the joint into flexion and extension. The knee joint is also capable of a slight internal and external rotation. The knee joint is the largest joint in the body and holds a lot of the body's weight. When an unbalanced force is applied to the knee joint, delicate ligaments that knit the joint together can become inflamed or begin to tear. There are four ligaments that are most common for injury. Those ligaments are: the anterior crutiate ligament (ACL), the posterior crutiate ligament (PCL), the medial crutiate ligament (MCL), and the lateral crutiate ligament (LCL). These ligaments attach to the femur and insert onto the tibia bone and work to keep the femur bone from sliding out of place. In addition to ligaments, the tendons of muscles come together to attach to or cross over the knee joint. These muscles are: the quadriceps, the hamstrings, the gastrocnemius, the gracilis, the sartorius, the popliteus, the plantaris muscle, and the soleus muscle. If the muscles surrounding the knee become tight, they can pull on the attachment sites located on the knee joint. This can cause pain in the knee area. In order to keep the knee joints healthy, a well-rounded yoga sequence that allows the knees to flex and extend will work to keep the knees functioning safely. Familiarize yourself with the bones and muscles of the knees to gain a deeper understanding of how the knees work.

KNEE JOINT

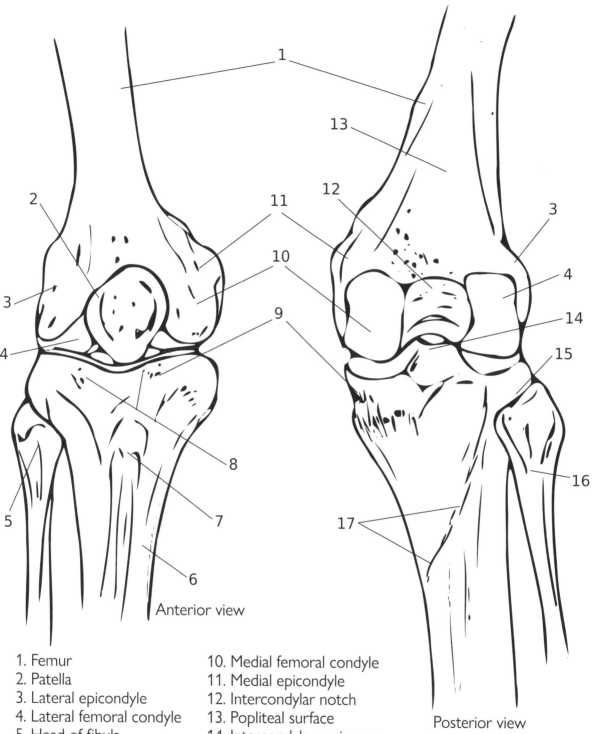

Anterior view

Posterior view

1. Femur
2. Patella
3. Lateral epicondyle
4. Lateral femoral condyle
5. Head of fibula
6. Tibia
7. Tibial tuberosity
8. Tibial plateau
9. Medial condyle

10. Medial femoral condyle
11. Medial epicondyle
12. Intercondylar notch
13. Popliteal surface
14. Intercondylar eminence
15. Tibiofibular joint
16. Neck of fibula
17. Soleal line

QUADRICEPS

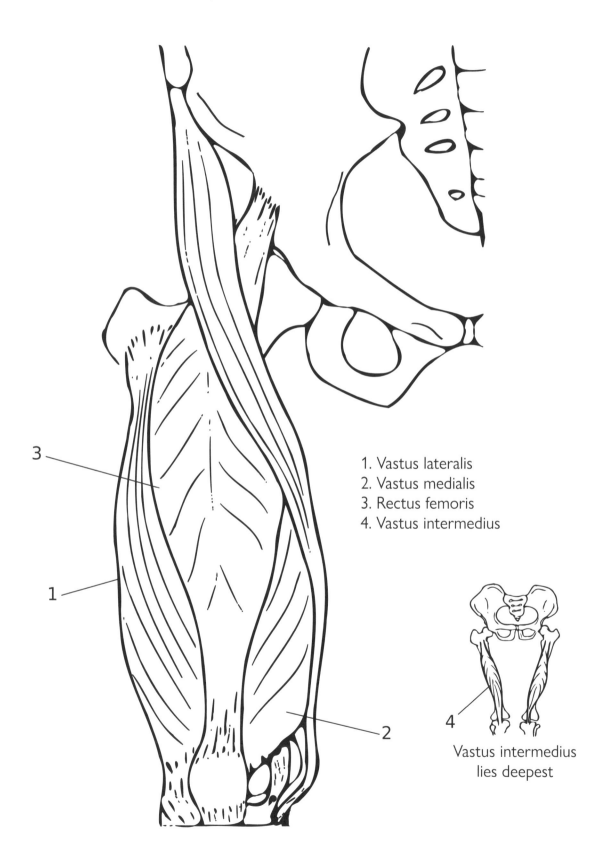

3

1

1. Vastus lateralis
2. Vastus medialis
3. Rectus femoris
4. Vastus intermedius

2

4

Vastus intermedius
lies deepest

HAMSTRINGS

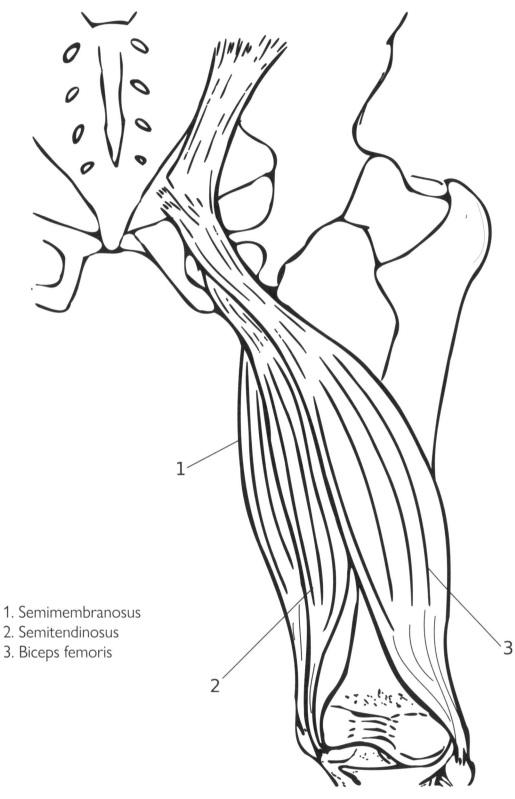

1. Semimembranosus
2. Semitendinosus
3. Biceps femoris

Posterior view of leg

KNEE FLEXION AND KNEE EXTENSION

Knee flexion and extension are movements created at the knee joint when muscles crossing the knee joint contract and relax. The knee flexor muscles contract to bring the knee into a bent position and the knee extensor muscles contract to straighten the leg at the knee joint. Having strong and balanced knee muscles helps stabilize the knee joint during movement, which can reduce the chance of knee injuries.

To activate the knee flexors

Grab a chair and put it behind you. From a standing position, let the edge of the chair touch your calves. Place your feet hip distance apart, keep your pelvis in a neutral position, and shift your weight to your left foot without sagging into your left hip joint. Lift your right foot off the floor and bend your knee. Let your calf muscle press up into the underside of the chair to engage the flexors of the knee. Hold that tension for 30 seconds then press your foot back into the floor. Repeat 3–5 times and switch legs.

What did you notice? Where did you feel the tension when you pressed your calf into the underside of the chair?

To activate the knee extensors

From a standing position, place your feet hip distance apart and shift your weight to your right leg without sagging into the hip joint. Straighten your left leg out in front of you and hover it a few inches off of the ground. Hold this position for 30 seconds. Repeat this movement 3–5 times and switch legs.

What did you notice? Did the extensor muscles in both knees begin to fatigue?

Practicing these small movements daily will bring strength and stability to your knee flexor and extensor muscles, which can decrease the chance of injury to the knee joint.

KNEE FLEXION AND KNEE EXTENSION

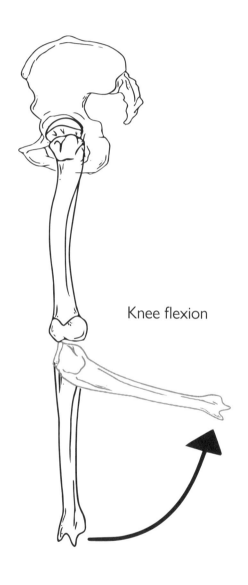

Knee flexion

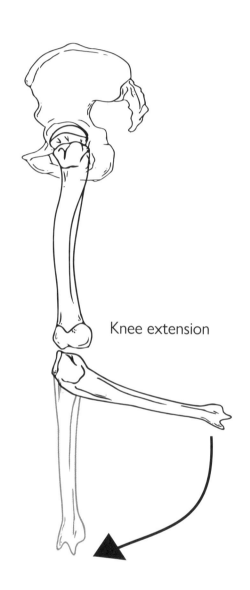

Knee extension

Knee Flexion
A movement that bends the knee and decreases the angle between the upper leg and lower leg

Knee Extension
A movement that extends the knee from a flexed position by increasing the angle between the upper leg and the lower leg

KNEE FLEXORS

The knee flexors are a group of muscles that contract to bring the knee into flexion, decreasing the angle between the upper leg and the lower leg. The muscles responsible for flexing the knee are the hamstrings: the biceps femoris, the semitendinosus, and the semimembranosus. Since the hamstring muscles originate on the posterior pelvis and attach to the knee, tight knee flexors can pull the pelvis down. When the pelvis is pulled down it is in a retroverted state (tucked), which flattens the lumbar curve of the spine. A flattened lumbar curve can put an unbalanced amount of stress onto the lower back and cause discomfort, pain and increased chance of injury to the spine. The pulling on the pelvis can lead to lower back pain. To lengthen the knee flexors, yoga poses or movements that bring the knees into extension can bring length to the hamstrings. It is important to ease into the extension of the knee by keeping the knees slightly bent in order to prevent over-lengthening or tearing. Weak hamstrings can create an unstable posterior pelvis and knee joint, which can increase the chances of injury. To strengthen the hamstrings, yoga poses or movements that bring the knees into flexion can bring strength to the knee flexor muscles. Virabhadrasana I and II (warrior I and II) and utkatasana konasana (goddess pose) bring flexion and strength to the knee flexors.

KNEE FLEXORS

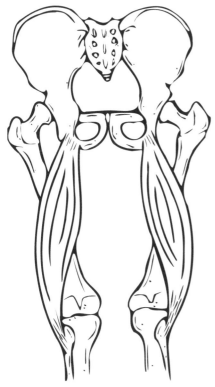

Rectus femoris

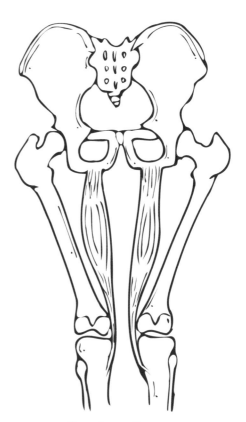

Semitendinosus

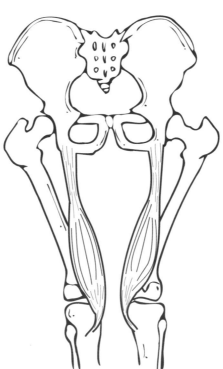

Semimembranosus

KNEE EXTENSORS

The knee extensors are a group of muscles that contract to extend the leg from a flexed position, increasing the angle between the upper leg and the lower leg. The muscles that produce this movement are the quadriceps: the rectus femoris, the vastus intermedius, the vastus lateralis, and the vastus medialis. When the muscles shorten and become tight, during flexion, the muscles can pull at the tendons of the muscle located on the anterior, lateral, and medial knee. To lengthen the quadriceps, poses or movements that bring the legs into slow and gentle flexion can work to bring length to the knee extensors. If the knee extensors become weak, the knee joint can become unstable during movement, which can increase the chances of injury. To strengthen the knee extensors, muscles that bring the knee into extension can bring strength to the muscles of extension. Vrksasana (tree pose), ardha chandrasana (half moon pose), and other standing poses can bring strength to the knee extensors.

KNEE EXTENSORS

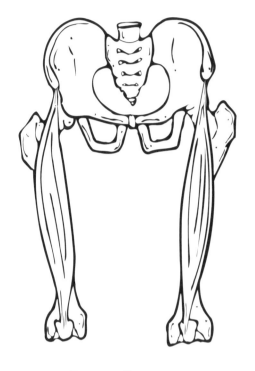

Rectus femoris

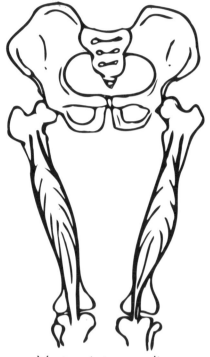

Vastus intermedius

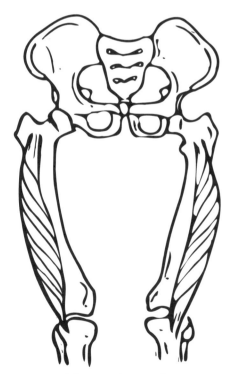

Vastus lateralis

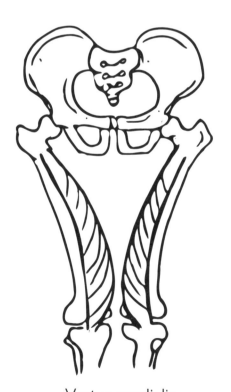

Vastus medialis

QUADRICEPS

The quadriceps are a group of four muscles located on the anterior portion of the thigh. When the fibers of these muscles contract, the knee joint extends. The quadriceps group consists of: the vastus lateralis, the vastus medialis, the vastus intermedius, and the rectus femoris. The quadriceps share an insertion point, coming together to create the quadriceps tendon. The quadriceps tendon inserts onto the superior patella (knee cap) and continues to form the patellar ligament. The patellar ligament starts from the inferior portion of the patella and inserts onto the tibial tuberosity of the tibia bone. When the quadriceps become overly tight, flexion of the knee can be limited and pain in the knee area can occur. To lengthen overly tight quadriceps, start off with poses that slightly flex and lengthen the muscles in order to prevent tearing the tendons at the attachment site of the knee. To prevent injury, make sure that the length of stretch comes from the middle of the quadriceps muscles instead of the knee joint.

Vastus lateralis: the vastus lateralis originates on the linea aspera and the greater trochanter of the femur bone. It extends down the lateral portion of the femur bone to insert into the patellar ligament and then crosses over the knee joint to insert onto the tibial tuberosity of the tibia bone. When the vastus lateralis becomes tight, lateral knee pain can occur.

Vastus medialis: the vastus medialis originates on the linea aspera and intertrochanteric line of the femur bone. It extends down the medial portion of the femur bone and inserts onto the tibial tuberosity of the tibia bone. Tightness of the vastus medialis can cause pain on the medial portion of the knee joint.

Vastus intermedius: the vastus intermedius sits deep on the femur bone. It originates on the anterior side of the femoral shaft and runs down the length of the anterior part of the femur bone to insert onto the tibial tuberosity.

Rectus femoris: the rectus femoris sits superficially to the other quadriceps muscles. Due to the origination on the anterior inferior iliac spine of the pelvis, when contracted, the rectus femoris is capable of producing two movements: extension of the knee joint and flexion of the hip joint. A tight rectus femoris can limit the ability to bring the knee into flexion or the hip into extension. When this muscle becomes too tight, pain in the anterior knee area can occur.

VASTUS LATERALIS

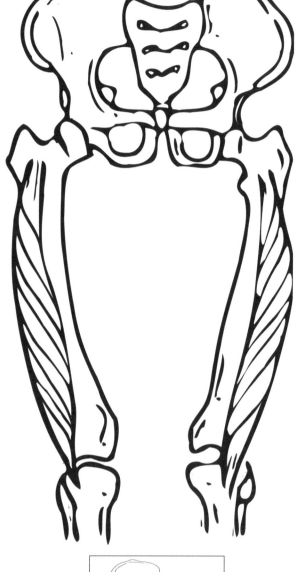

Action: Extension of the leg at the knee joint

Origin: Linea aspera and greater trochanter of femur

Insertion: Patellar ligament and tibial tuberosity

Agonists: Vastus medialis, vastus intermedius, rectus femoris

Antagonists: Biceps femoris, semitendinosus, semimembranosus

Poses: *Contracts:* uttanasana, adho mukha svanasana. *Lengthens:* supta baddah konasana, setu bandhasana

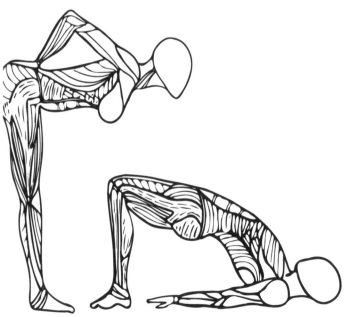

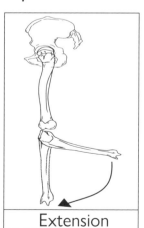

Extension

VASTUS MEDIALIS

Action: Extension of the leg at the knee joint

Origin: Linea aspera and intertrochanteric line

Insertion: Tibial tuberosity

Agonists: Vastus intermedius, vastus lateralis, rectus femoris

Antagonists: Biceps femoris, semitendinosus, semimembranosus

Poses: *Contracts:* adho mukha svanasana, uttanasana, dandasana. *Lengthens:* supta baddah konasana, Lord Shiva's dancing pose (flexed leg)

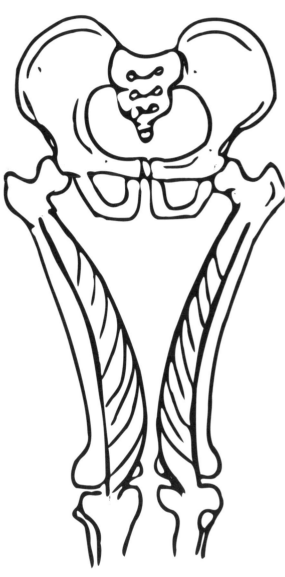

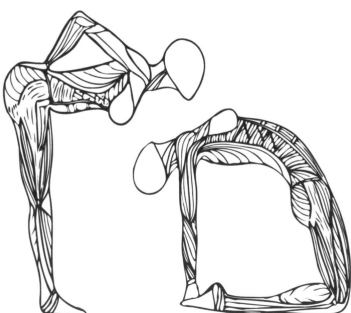

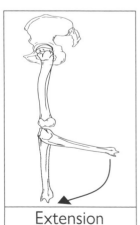

Extension

VASTUS INTERMEDIUS

Action: Extension of the leg at the knee joint

Origin: Anterior side of femoral shaft

Insertion: Tibial tuberosity

Agonists: Vastus medialis, vastus lateralis, vastus femoris

Antagonists: Biceps femoris, semitendinosus, semimembranosus

Poses: *Contracts:* uttanasana, dandasana, utthita trikonasana. *Lengthens:* ustrasana, supta virasana, bakasana, malasana

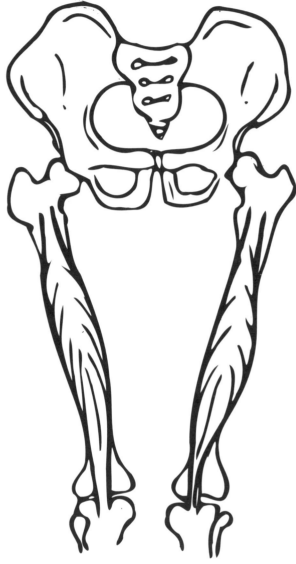

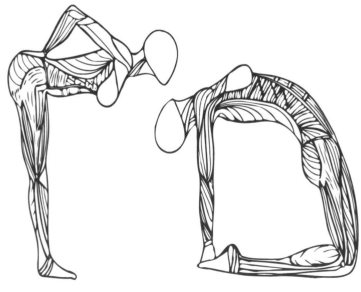

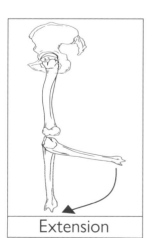

Extension

RECTUS FEMORIS

Action: Flexion of the hip joint, extension of the knee joint

Origin: Anterior inferior iliac spine of the pelvis and acetabular roof of hip joint

Insertion: Tibial tuberosity

Agonists: *Flexion:* iliopsoas. *Extension:* vastus intermedius, vastus lateralis, vastus medialis

Antagonists: *Flexion:* gluteus maximus, semitendinosus, semimembranosus, biceps femoris, adductor magnus. *Extension:* biceps femoris, semitendinosus, semimembranosus

Poses: *Contracts:* uttanasana, adho mukha svanasana. *Lengthens:* ustrasana, urdhva dhanurasana

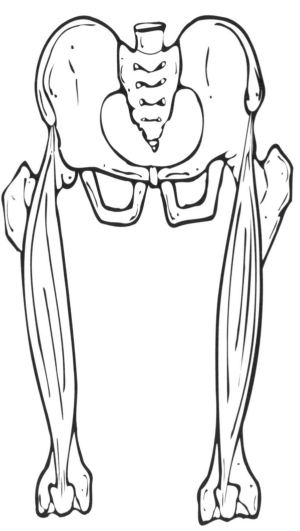

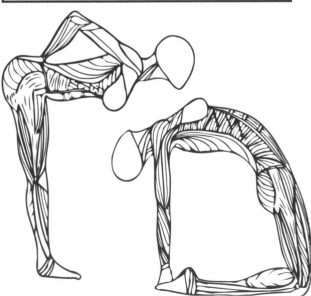

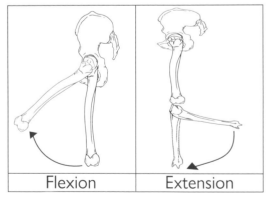

Flexion   Extension

HAMSTRINGS

The hamstrings are a group of three muscles located on the posterior thigh. The hamstring muscles contract to bring the knee joint into flexion or the hip joint into extension. The three muscles that make up the hamstrings are: the semimembranosus, the semitendinosus, and the biceps femoris.

Semimembranosus: the semimembranosus sits medially on the femur bone and originates on the posterior lateral surface of the ischial tuberosity. It extends down the length of the femur bone and crosses over the knee joint to insert onto the superior medial condyle of the tibia.

Semitendinosus: the semitendinosus sits in between the semimembranosus and biceps femoris. It originates on the posterior surface of the ischial tuberosity and runs down the length of the posterior femur bone to join tendons with the gracilis and sartorius.

Biceps femoris: the biceps femoris originates on the posterior surface of the ischial tuberosity and the lateral lip of the linea aspera of the femur bone.

SEMIMEMBRANOSUS

Action: Extension of leg at hip, flexion of knee joint, internal rotation of knee when flexed, pelvic stabilization

Origin: Posterior lateral surface of ischial tuberosity and sacrotuberous ligament

Insertion: Superior medial condyle of tibia, popliteal ligament

Agonists: *Extension:* gluteus maximus, semitendinosus, biceps femoris (LH), adductor magnus. *Flexion:* biceps femoris, semitendinosus. *Internal rotation:* semitendinosus, popliteus

Antagonists: *Extension:* psoas major, iliacus. *Flexion:* vastus lateralis, vastus medialis, vastus intermedius, rectus femoris. *Internal rotation:* biceps femoris

Poses: *Contracts:* virabhadrasana III, dhanurasana, salabhasana. *Lengthens:* hanumasana, utthita trikonasana

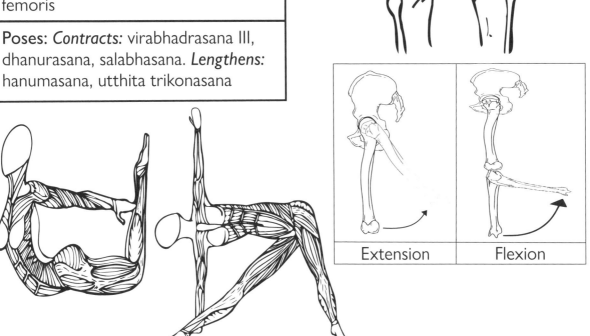

Extension | Flexion

SEMITENDINOSUS

Action: Extension of the leg at hip, flexion of knee joint, internal rotation of knee when flexed

Origin: Posterior surface of ischial tuberosity

Insertion: Medial tibial condyle, popliteal ligament with fibers inserting into popliteal fascia

Agonists: *Extension:* gluteus maximus, semitendinosus, biceps femoris (LH), adductor magnus. *Flexion:* biceps femoris, semitendinosus. *Internal rotation:* semitendinosus, popliteus

Antagonists: *Extension:* psoas major, iliacus. *Flexion:* vastus lateralis, vastus medialis, vastus intermedius, rectus femoris. *Internal rotation:* biceps femoris

Poses: *Contracts:* shalambasana, utkatasana, dhanurasana. *Lengthens:* hanumasana, prasarita padottanasana, utthita trikonasana, adho mukha svanasana

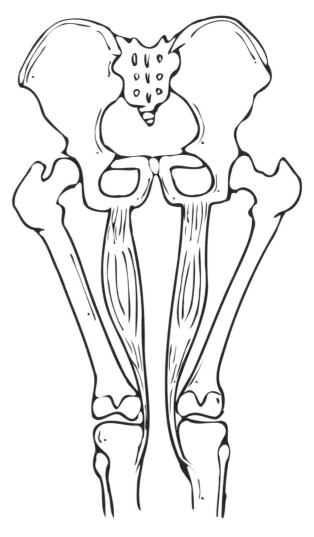

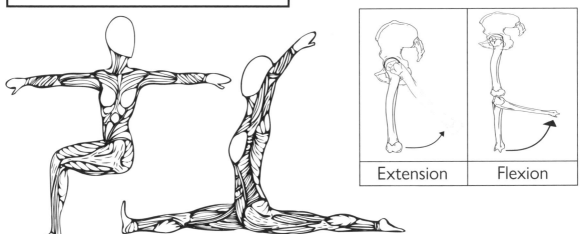

Extension | Flexion

BICEPS FEMORIS

Action: Flexion of knee joint. Extension of leg at hip. Slight internal rotation when knee is flexed

Origin: Posterior surface of ischial tuberosity (LH), lateral lip of linea aspera on middle third of femur (SH)

Insertion: Head of fibula

Agonists: *Flexion:* semitendinosus, semimembranosus. *Extension of thigh at hip:* gluteus maximus, semitendinosus, semimembranosus, adductor magnus

Antagonists: *Flexion:* vastus lateralis, vastus medialis, vastus intermedius, rectus femoris. *Extension of thigh at hip:* iliopsoas

Poses: *Contracts:* utkatasana. *Lengthens:* hanumasana

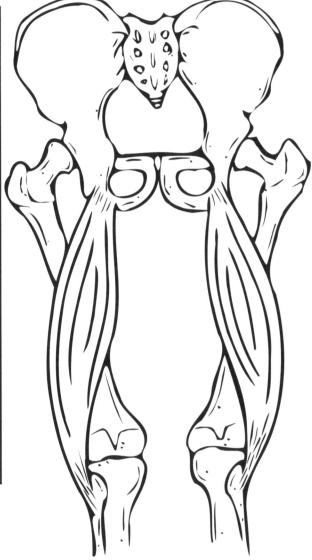

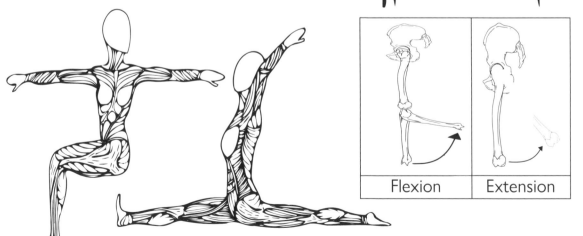

Flexion | Extension

LOWER LEG ANATOMY

The lower leg consists of the tibia, the fibula, the ankle joint, and the foot. The muscles that make up the lower leg contract to dorsiflex, plantarflex, invert, and evert the ankle joint. They also contract to flex and extend the toes. The anterior tibialis is located on the anterior lower leg and is a strong muscle that dorsiflexes the ankle joint, which is seen in yoga poses that require the toes to point upwards. The gastrocnemius and soleus muscles come together to insert onto the posterior portion of the calcaneus, or heel bone. This tendon of insertion is commonly known as the "Achilles tendon." These muscles are responsible for plantarflexing the ankle, which is seen in yoga poses that require the toes to point or press into the floor.

TIBIA AND FIBULA

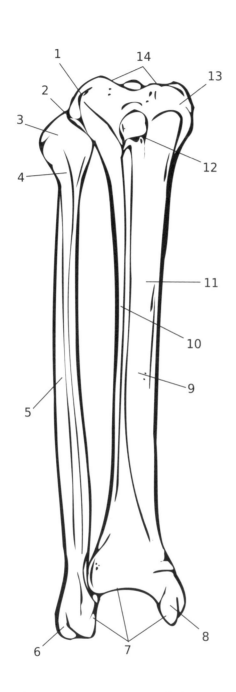
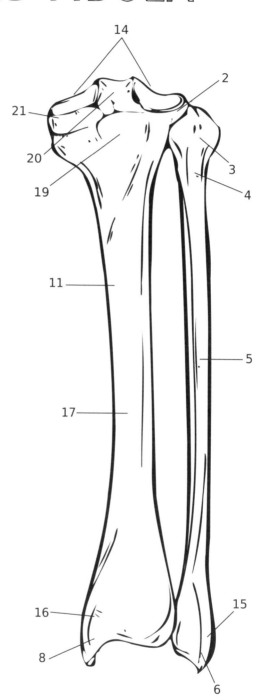

1. Lateral condyle
2. Tibiofibular joint
3. Head of fibula
4. Neck of fibula
5. Fibula shaft
6. Lateral malleolus
7. Ankle mortise

8. Medial malleolus
9. Medial surface
10. Lateral surface
11. Tibia shaft
12. Tibial tuberosity
13. Medial condyle
14. Tibial plateau

15. Lateral malleolar fossa
16. Malleolar groove
17. Posterior surface
18. Soleal line
19. Head of tibia
20. Intercondylar eminence
21. Medial condyle

MUSCLES OF THE LOWER LEG

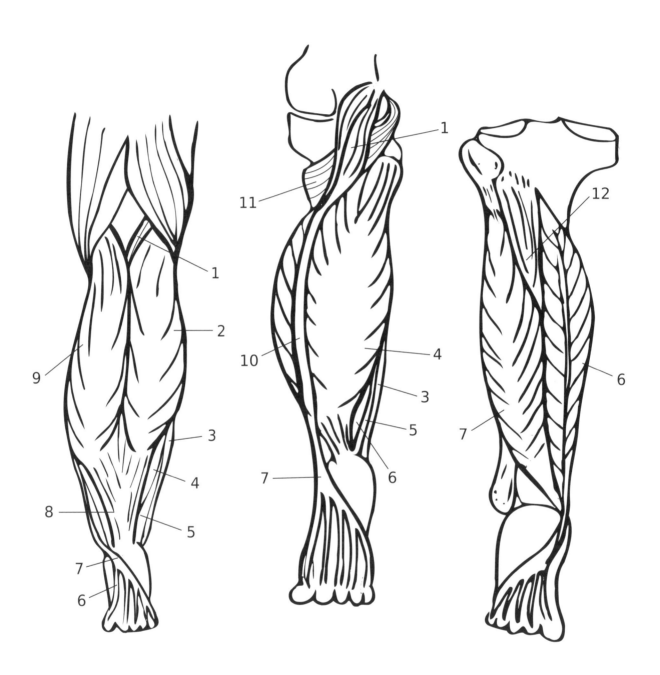

1. Plantaris
2. Gastrocnemius (lateral head)
3. Fibularis brevis
4. Soleus
5. Fibularis longus
6. Flexor hallucis longus
7. Flexor digitorum longus
8. Achilles tendon
9. Gastrocnemius (medial head)
10. Plantaris tendon
11. Popliteus
12. Tibialis posterior

MUSCLES OF THE LOWER LEG

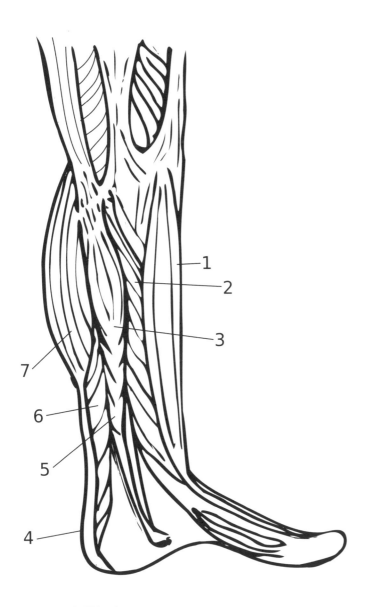

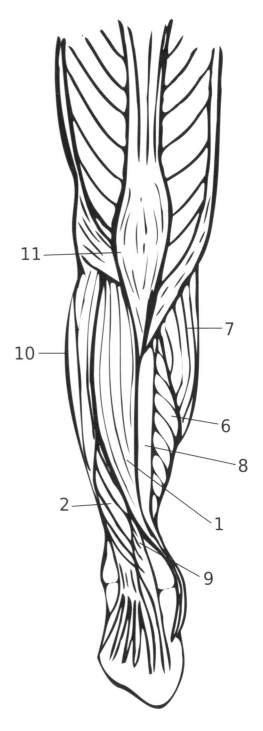

1. Tibialis anterior
2. Extensor digitorum longus
3. Fibularis longus
4. Achilles tendon
5. Fibularis brevis
6. Soleus
7. Gastrocnemius
8. Tibia shaft
9. Extensor hallucis longus
10. Fibularis longus
11. Tibial tuberosity

THE SHOULDER JOINT

The shoulder area consists of three bones that come together to create four joints on the posterior lateral sides of the ribcage. The three bones that make up the shoulder area are: the scapula (shoulder blade), the clavicle (collar bone), and the humerus bone (upper arm bone). Together those bones create articulations with each other and the ribcage to allow for movement of the shoulders and arms.

Scapula: the scapula is a flat triangular-shaped bone that provides stability during movements of the arm.

Clavicle: the clavicle is an s-shaped bone that forms an articulation with the sternum and the acromion of the scapula.

Humerus: the humerus is the upper bone of the arm. The head of the humerus sits in the glenoid cavity of the scapula to create the shoulder joint.

The joints created by the three shoulder bones are: the glenohumeral joint, the acromioclavicular joint (AC joint), the sternoclavicular joint (SC joint), and the scapulothoracic joint.

Glenohumeral joint: more commonly known as the shoulder joint, the glenohumeral joint is the articulation created between the glenoid cavity of the scapula and the head of the humerus bone. The glenohumeral joint is a highly moveable ball-and-socket joint that allows for a wide range of movements.

Acromioclavicular joint: the AC joint is the articulation created between the acromion of the scapula and the distal end of the clavicle.

Sternoclavicular joint: the SC joint is the articulation created between the sternum and proximal side of the clavicle.

Scapulothoracic joint: the scapulothoracic joint is the articulation created between the scapula and the ribcage and is the site of scapular protraction, retraction, upward rotation, and downward rotation.

At the sites of articulation, ligaments expand to attach bone to bone and hold the bones steady. The joints are then surrounded in muscles that provide stability and movement to the shoulder area. If the muscles of the shoulder become weak, their ability to stabilize the shoulder joints decreases. This can put undue stress onto the ligaments. Since the ligaments are not designed to hold a lot of weight, the ligaments can tear from the bone, resulting in a shoulder injury. To make sure the shoulder muscles are strong and stable, it is important to create a yoga flow that includes all of the shoulder movements. The movements that the shoulder can produce are: abduction, adduction, internal rotation, external rotation, flexion, extension, protraction, retraction, upward rotation, downward rotation, elevation, and depression.

SHOULDER

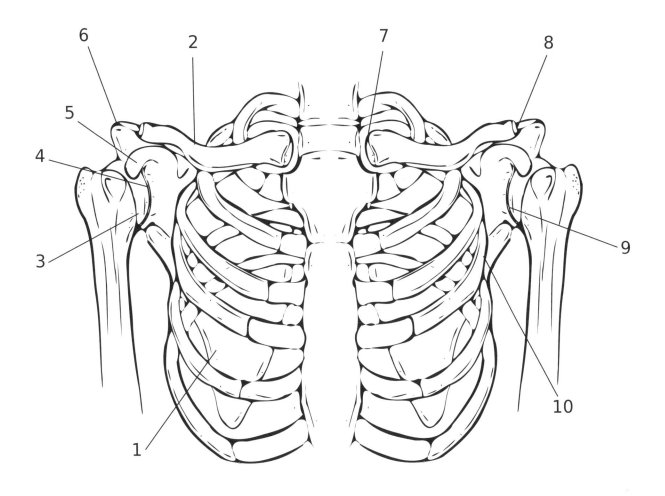

1. Scapula
2. Clavicle
3. Head of humerus
4. Glenoid cavity
5. Coracoid process
6. Acromion
7. Sternoclavicular joint
8. Acromioclavicular joint
9. Glenohumeral joint
10. Scapulothoracic joint

SCACPULA

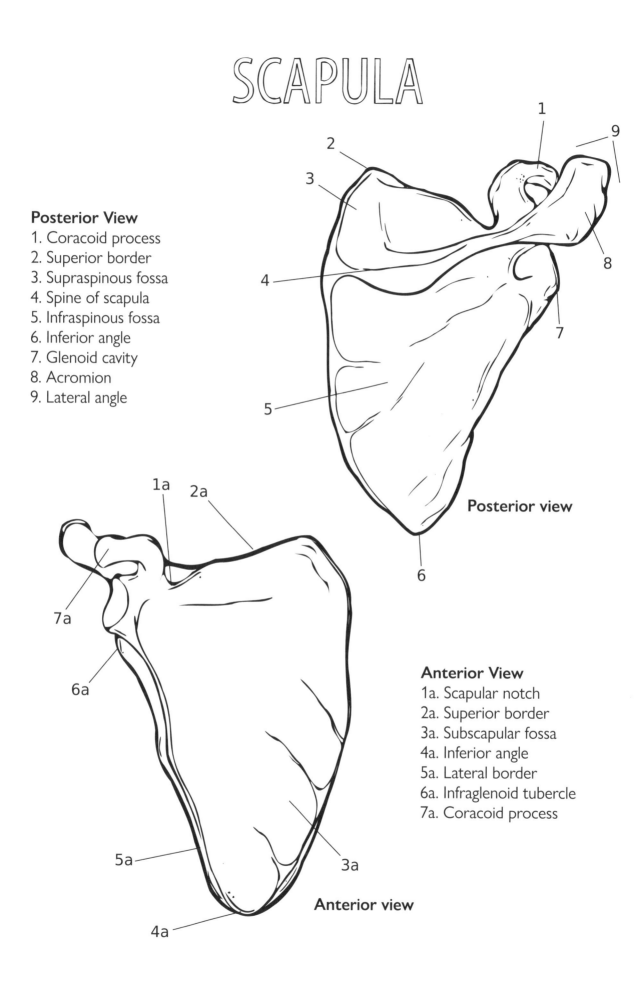

Posterior View
1. Coracoid process
2. Superior border
3. Supraspinous fossa
4. Spine of scapula
5. Infraspinous fossa
6. Inferior angle
7. Glenoid cavity
8. Acromion
9. Lateral angle

2

3

1

9

4

8

7

5

Posterior view

6

1a   2a

7a

6a

Anterior View
1a. Scapular notch
2a. Superior border
3a. Subscapular fossa
4a. Inferior angle
5a. Lateral border
6a. Infraglenoid tubercle
7a. Coracoid process

3a

5a

Anterior view

4a

SCAPULA AND CLAVICLE

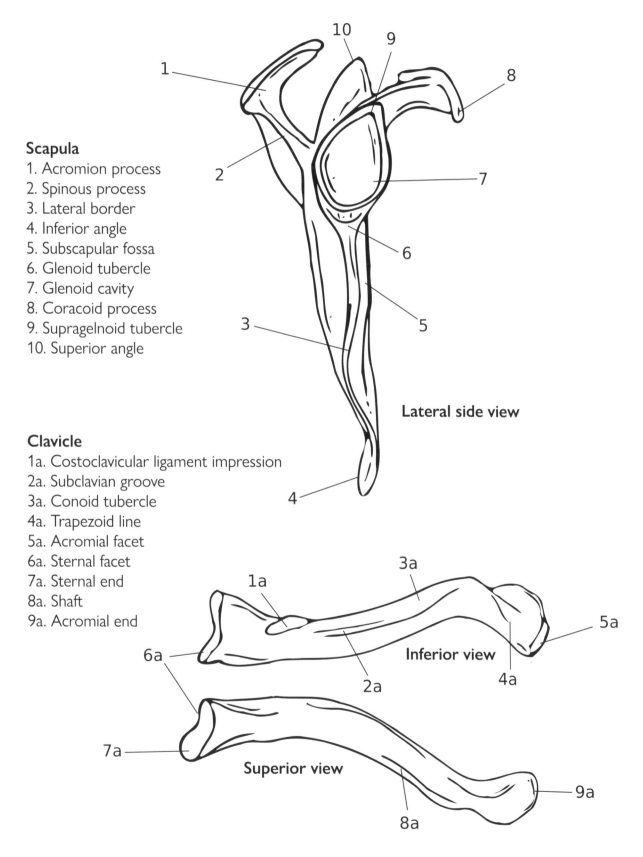

Scapula

1. Acromion process
2. Spinous process
3. Lateral border
4. Inferior angle
5. Subscapular fossa
6. Glenoid tubercle
7. Glenoid cavity
8. Coracoid process
9. Supragelnoid tubercle
10. Superior angle

Lateral side view

Clavicle

1a. Costoclavicular ligament impression
2a. Subclavian groove
3a. Conoid tubercle
4a. Trapezoid line
5a. Acromial facet
6a. Sternal facet
7a. Sternal end
8a. Shaft
9a. Acromial end

Inferior view

Superior view

HUMERUS

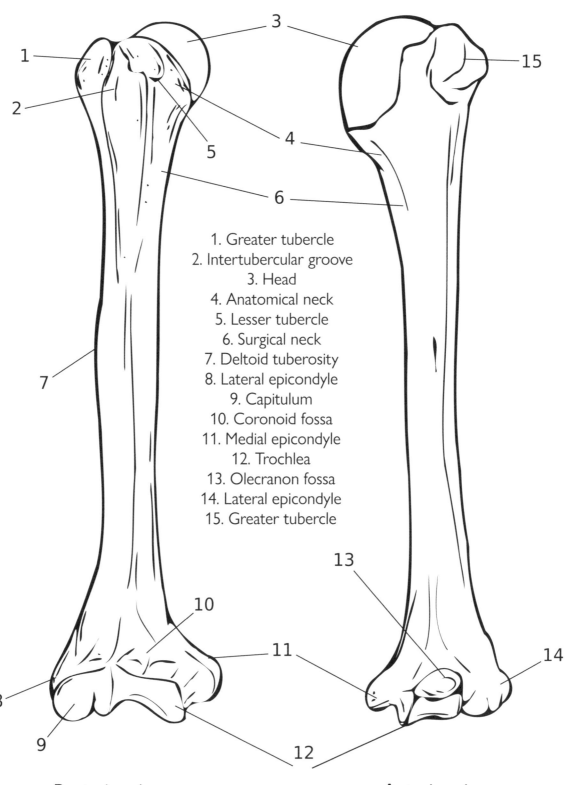

1. Greater tubercle
2. Intertubercular groove
3. Head
4. Anatomical neck
5. Lesser tubercle
6. Surgical neck
7. Deltoid tuberosity
8. Lateral epicondyle
9. Capitulum
10. Coronoid fossa
11. Medial epicondyle
12. Trochlea
13. Olecranon fossa
14. Lateral epicondyle
15. Greater tubercle

Posterior view

Anterior view

POSTERIOR MUSCLES

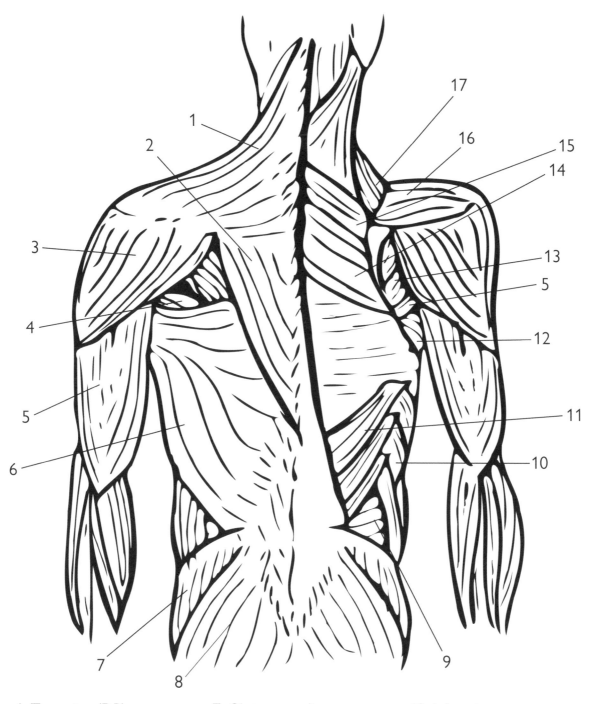

1. Trapezius (DP)
2. Trapezius (AP)
3. Deltoid (PF)
4. Teres major
5. Triceps brachii
6. Latissimus dorsi

7. Gluteus medius
8. Gluteus maximus
9. Internal oblique
10. External oblique
11. Serratus posterior
12. Serratus anterior

13. Infraspinatus
14. Rhomboid major
15. Rhomboid minor
16. Supraspinatus
17. Levator scapulae

SHOULDER MUSCLES

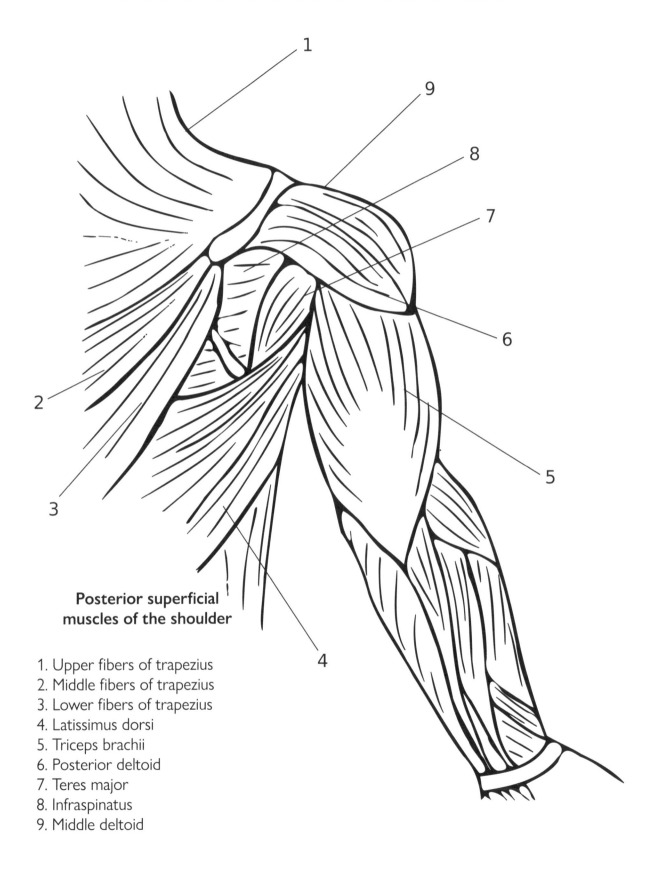

Posterior superficial muscles of the shoulder

1. Upper fibers of trapezius
2. Middle fibers of trapezius
3. Lower fibers of trapezius
4. Latissimus dorsi
5. Triceps brachii
6. Posterior deltoid
7. Teres major
8. Infraspinatus
9. Middle deltoid

SHOULDER MUSCLES

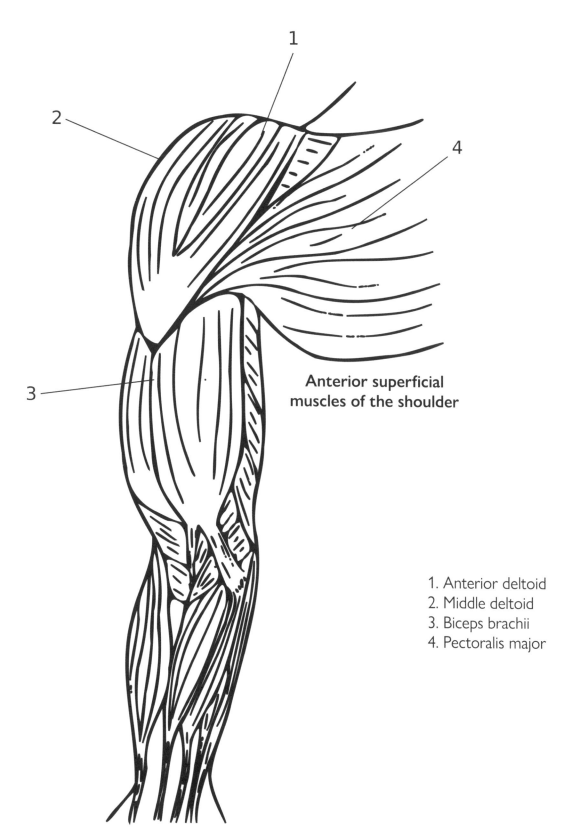

1

2

4

3

Anterior superficial muscles of the shoulder

1. Anterior deltoid
2. Middle deltoid
3. Biceps brachii
4. Pectoralis major

SHOULDER ABDUCTION AND SHOULDER ADDUCTION

The muscles of shoulder abduction and adduction are referred to as "shoulder abductors" and "shoulder adductors." These muscles contract and relax to bring the humerus bones away from (shoulder abduction) or towards (shoulder adduction) the midline of the body. Since the shoulder joint is the most mobile joint in the body, it is important to strengthen and lengthen the shoulder abductors and adductors in order to bring stability to the shoulder joint. Stabilizing the shoulder joints will increase the longevity of the joints and reduce the chance of injury.

To activate the shoulder abductors

Stand in mountain pose in a doorway with your palms facing in towards your thighs. Keep your pelvis neutral and slightly engage your abdominals for thoracic stability. Stabilize the shoulder blades onto the back of the ribcage. Begin to lift your arms away from your body towards the door jamb. Press the back of your hands into the door jamb to activate the shoulder abductor muscles. Hold the tension for 30 seconds. Repeat 3–5 times.

What did you notice? Did your shoulder joint feel more stable and strong when you consciously stabilized your shoulder blade onto the back of your ribcage before lifting your arms? Now try to keep that stability in the shoulder blades while abducting your arms without the door jamb. Are you able to use the shoulder joints to stabilize and support the weight of your arms?

To activate the shoulder adductors

Stand in mountain pose with your palms touching the outside of your thighs. Keep your pelvis neutral and slightly engage your abdominals for thoracic stability. Stabilize your shoulder blades onto the back of your ribcage. Press your upper arm bones into your ribcage. Hold this tension for 30 seconds. Repeat 3–5 times.

What did you notice? Was it harder than you expected? Did you feel the muscles in the shoulder area working?

Practice these movements daily to bring strength and stability to the most mobile joint in the body, the shoulder.

Note: Stabilizing your shoulder blades onto the back of your ribcage helps the muscles of the scapulothoracic joint activate and provides support and stability to the shoulder joint as the arms move.

SHOULDER ABDUCTION AND SHOULDER ADDUCTION

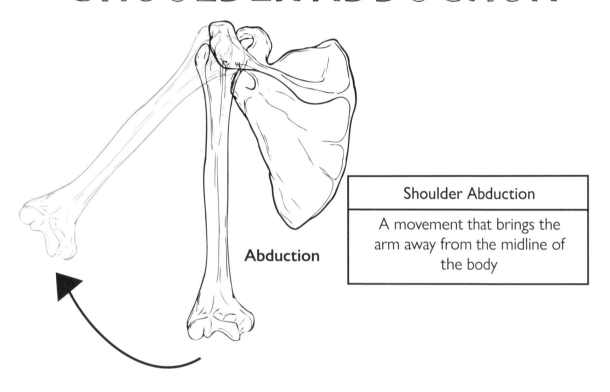

Abduction

Shoulder Abduction
A movement that brings the arm away from the midline of the body

Shoulder Adduction
A movement that brings the arm in toward or across the midline of the body

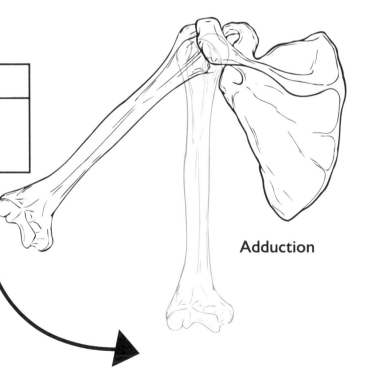

Adduction

SHOULDER ABDUCTORS

The shoulder abductors are a group of muscles that contract to bring the arm away from the midline of the body. The muscles that produce this movement are: the biceps brachii, the middle deltoids, the serratus anterior, and the supraspinatus. The shoulder joint is a highly moveable joint, and without activities that take the shoulders through the full range of movements, the muscles can become weak and the joint unstable. An unstable joint can eventually lead to injury. To prevent injury, strengthen weak shoulder abductors by participating in yoga poses or movements that abduct the arm out to the side. Vasisthasana (side plank pose) is a great pose that helps strengthen the abductors of the shoulder. If the abductors become too tight, they can throw off the balance between movements of the shoulder and can also eventually produce discomfort. To lengthen the muscles of the shoulder, yoga poses or movements that require the arm to adduct back towards or across the midline of the body will help.

SHOULDER ABDUCTORS

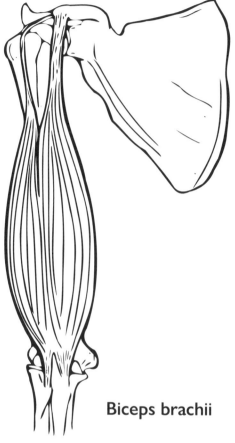

Biceps brachii

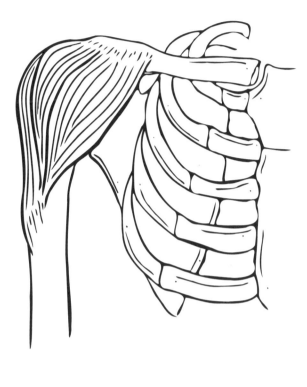

Deltoid (middle fibers)

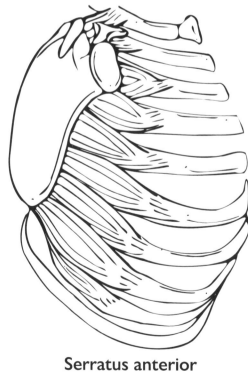

Serratus anterior

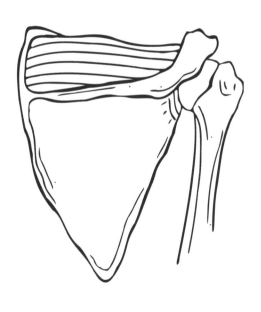

Supraspinatus

SHOULDER ADDUCTORS

The shoulder adductors are a group of muscles that contract to bring the arms back in towards the body or across the midline of the body. The muscles responsible for shoulder adduction are: the pectoralis major, the latissimus dorsi, the teres major, and the triceps brachii. Overly tight shoulder adductors can throw off the balance of the shoulder joint and increase risk of injury. To lengthen the shortened muscles, participating in yoga poses or movements that require the arms to abduct away from the body will help bring length to those muscles. If shoulder adductors are weak, limited use of the shoulder can occur as well as increased chances of injury. To strengthen the shoulder adductors, participating in yoga poses or movements that adduct the arms inward towards the body will help bring strength to those muscles. Kumbhakasana (plank pose) and forearm plank pose will help strengthen the shoulder adductors since they require a slight adduction of the arms.

SHOULDER ADDUCTORS

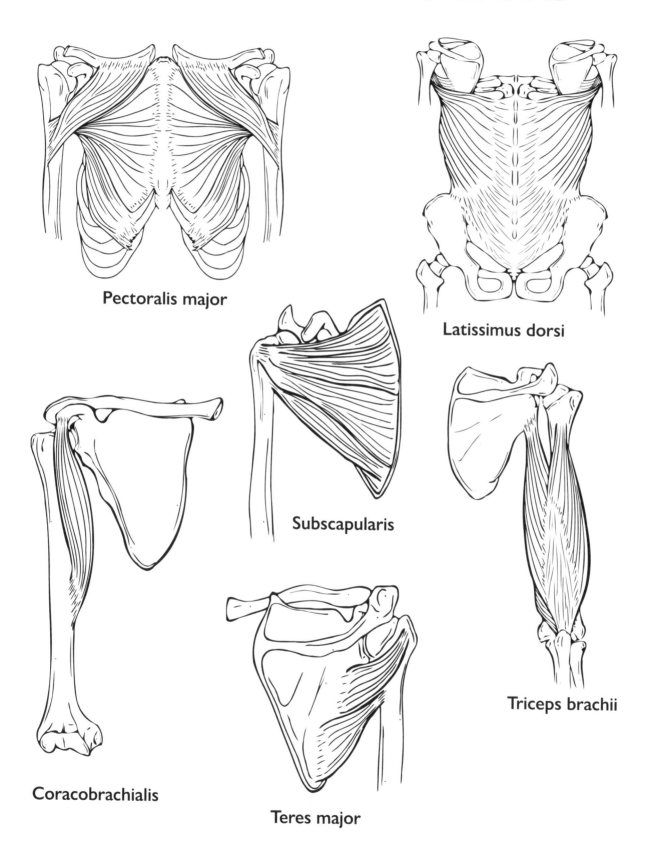

Pectoralis major

Latissimus dorsi

Subscapularis

Coracobrachialis

Teres major

Triceps brachii

EXTERNAL AND INTERNAL SHOULDER ROTATION

External and internal rotation of the shoulder occurs when muscles contract and relax to rotate the humerus bone away from or towards the midline of the body. Theses muscles are referred to as "external rotators" and "internal rotators" of the shoulder. Bringing strength and length to these muscle groups helps stabilize the shoulder joint and reduce the chance of injury to the shoulder joint.

To activate the external rotators of the shoulder
Standing in mountain position with the palms facing the thighs, stabilize the shoulder blades at the scapulothoracic joint. With the origin of movement beginning in the shoulder joint, rotate the humerus bone outwards away from the midline of the body so the palms are now facing away from the thighs. Hold for 1–5 seconds and then release back to resting position. Repeat 3–5 times.

What did you notice? Did you feel any spots of tension?

To activate the internal rotators of the shoulder
Standing in mountain pose with the palms facing forwards, stabilize the shoulder blades at the scapulothoracic joint. Then, by initiating movement at shoulder joint, begin to rotate the humerus bone in towards the midline of the body so that the palms face behind you. Hold for 1–5 seconds and release back to resting position. Repeat 3–5 times.

What did you notice? Were there any sticky movements? Or did your shoulder joint move smoothly?

Practicing these movements daily will allow the rotators of the shoulder joint to build strength to provide stability.

Note: In order to fully activate the rotators of the shoulders and to prevent injury from an unbalanced movement of torque, it is important for the origin of the movement to begin within the shoulder joint and to rotate down the humerus bone to the lower arm and wrist, rather than the movement originating at the wrist and rotating up the lower arm bone and humerus into the shoulder.

EXTERNAL AND INTERNAL SHOULDER ROTATION

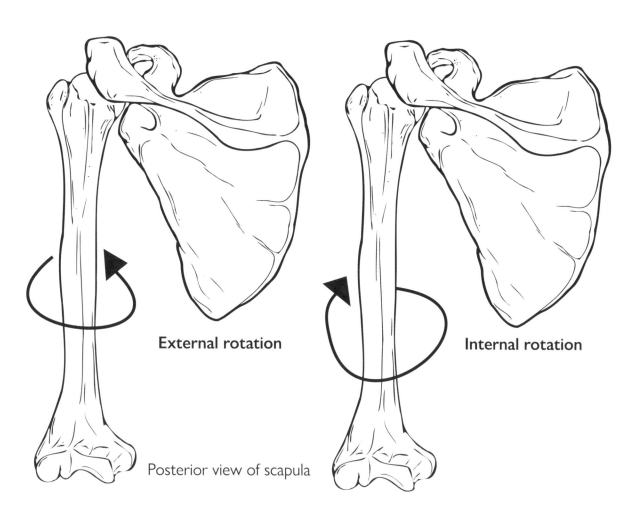

External rotation

Posterior view of scapula

Internal rotation

External Shoulder Rotation
A movement that rotates the arm away from the midline of the body

Internal Shoulder Rotation
A movement that rotates the arm towards the midline of the body

EXTERNAL ROTATORS OF THE SHOULDER

The external rotators are a group of muscles that contract to rotate the arm away from the midline of the body. The mucles responsible for this action are: the posterior deltoids, the infraspinatus, the supraspinatus, and the teres minor. With a poor, slouching posture, the arms tend to roll forwards into internal rotation. While the arm continues to internally rotate, the external rotators become less active and weak—creating a vicious cycle of bad posture. To rid the habit of slouching forwards into internal rotation, lengthening the internal rotators and strengthening the external rotators can help achieve this goal. As the external rotators become stronger, the integrity of the shoulder joint begins to come back to life. Some yoga poses that strengthen the external rotators are adho mukha svanasana (downward facing dog) and virabhadrasana II (warrior II) with palms facing up towards the ceiling. Bringing awareness to the state of your shoulder blades during inactivity will help identify postural habits while creating a stronger mind–body connection with the external rotators of the shoulder.

EXTERNAL ROTATORS
OF THE SHOULDER

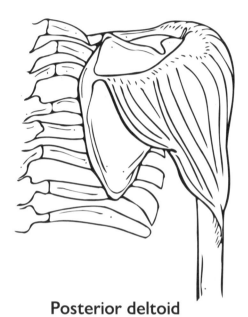

Posterior deltoid

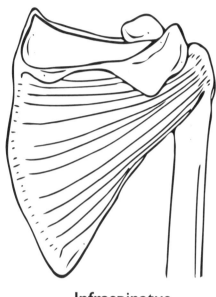

Infraspinatus

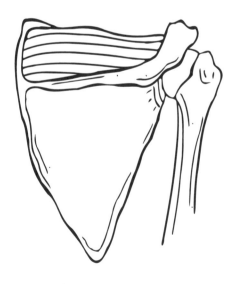

Supraspinatus

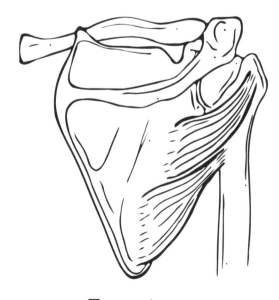

Teres minor

INTERNAL ROTATORS OF THE SHOULDER

The internal rotators of the shoulder are a group of muscles that contract to rotate the arm inwards towards the midline of the body. These muscles are: the pectoralis major, the biceps brachii, the anterior deltoid, the subscapularis, the latissimus dorsi, and the teres major. Poor posture can contribute to tightened and shortened shoulder internal rotator muscles. When these muscles consistently contract to support the slouching of bad posture, it throws off the balance of the rest of the muscles in the shoulder.

The external rotators may become weak and the stability of the shoulders can weaken as well. And since the shoulder joint is a highly moveable joint, it is important to maintain balance in the shoulder blades in all areas of movement. In order to counteract and lengthen the muscles of internal rotation, yoga poses and movements that allow the arm to externally rotate away from the midline of the body will help achieve length. Some poses that bring the arm into external rotation are adho mukha svanasana (downward facing dog) and balasana (child's pose) with palms facing towards the ceiling.

Once the internal rotators are lengthened and brought back into balance, yoga poses that bring the arm into internal rotation can help strengthen these muscles. Some poses that bring the arm into internal rotation are garudasana (eagle pose) and paschima namaskarasana (reverse prayer pose). The first step to lengthening and strengthening the internal rotators are to become aware of the movement inside the body.

INTERNAL ROTATORS OF THE SHOULDER

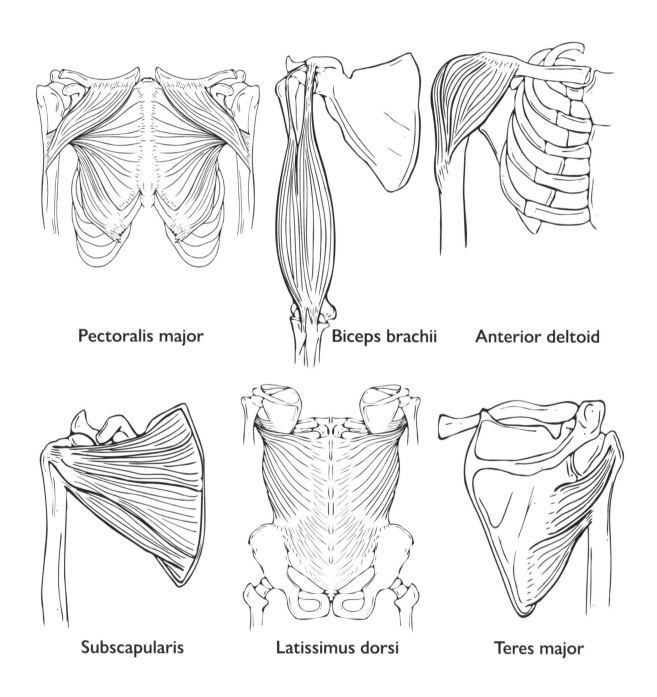

Pectoralis major

Biceps brachii

Anterior deltoid

Subscapularis

Latissimus dorsi

Teres major

SHOULDER FLEXION AND SHOULDER EXTENSION

Shoulder flexion and extension are movements that occur when muscles contract and relax to bring the humerus bone forwards (shoulder flexion) or backward (shoulder extension) in space. These movements can be seen when entering into virabhadrasana I (warrior I) or when putting the arms back for ardha purvottanasana (reverse table top pose). Known as the "shoulder flexors" and "shoulder extensors," these muscles also help to bring stability to the shoulder joint, which help reduce the chance of injury to the shoulder joint.

To activate the shoulder flexors
Standing in mountain pose with your palms facing your thighs, neutralize the pelvis and slightly engage the abdominals for thoracic stability. Stabilize the scapulothoracic joint. Begin to lift both arms forwards and above your head without jutting the ribcage forwards. Hold for 30 seconds.

What did you notice about your shoulder blades as you lifted your arms? Can you feel how they are moving?

To activate the shoulder extensors
Standing in mountain pose with your palms facing your thighs, neutralize your spine and slightly engage the abdominals for thoracic stability. Stabilize your scapulothoracic joint. Begin to press your arms back behind you as far as you can without feeling pain. Hold for 30 seconds.

What did you notice? Is this movement easy and normal or difficult and foreign? Can you feel how your shoulder blades are moving when you press your shoulders back?

Couple these movements and repeat 5–10 times.

Note: As the shoulder flexes the arm forwards and above the head, the shoulder blades depress down the back and protract outwards from the midline of the body. As the shoulder extends the arms down and backwards, the shoulder blades elevate and retract in towards the midline.

SHOULDER FLEXION AND SHOULDER EXTENSION

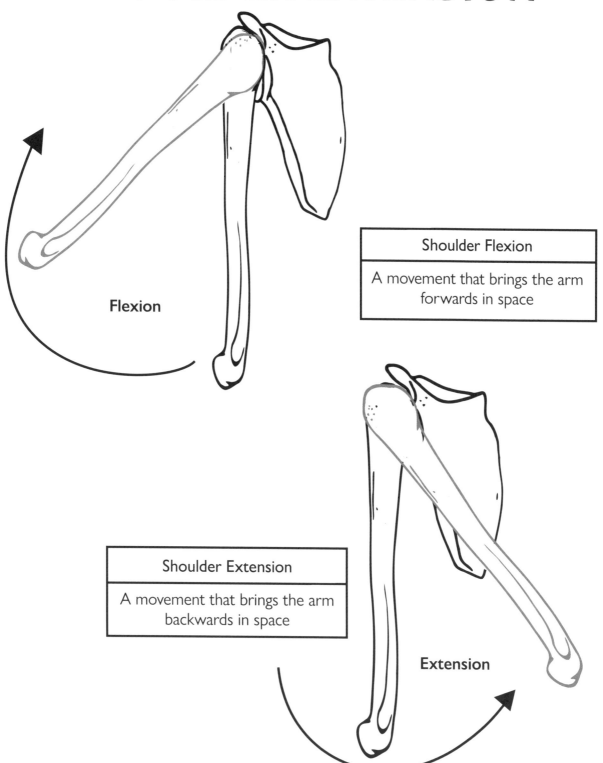

Flexion

Shoulder Flexion
A movement that brings the arm forwards in space

Shoulder Extension
A movement that brings the arm backwards in space

Extension

SHOULDER FLEXORS

The flexors of the shoulders are a group of muscles that contract to bring the arms forwards in space. The shoulders flex when the arms reach out to grab something or are raised over the head. The muscles that work together to produce shoulder flexion are: the anterior deltoid, the biceps brachii, the coracobrachialis, and the pectoralis major. When the shoulder flexors become overly tight, an inability to produce deep shoulder extension may occur. This can also lead to weakened shoulder extensors. In order to lengthen the shoulder flexors, participating in yoga poses like purvottanasana (reverse plank) and ustrasana (camel pose) or movements that bring the arm into extension at the shoulder joint can work to bring length to the shoulder flexion muscles. If the shoulder flexors become overly inactive, ability to lift heavy objects may decrease and chances of injury may increase. To bring strength to the shoulder flexors, yoga poses and movements that bring the arm forwards in space will help bring strength to these muscles. Some poses that bring strength to the shoulder flexors are kumbhakasana (plank pose) and adho mukha svanasana (downward facing dog).

SHOULDER FLEXORS

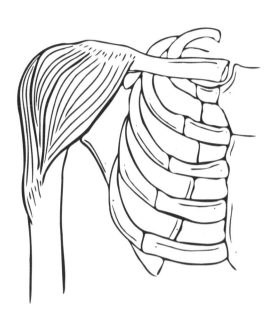

Anterior deltoid

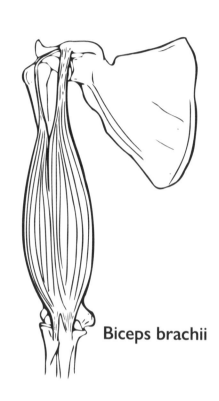

Biceps brachii

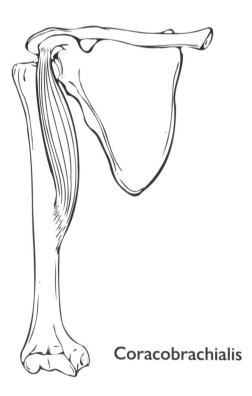

Coracobrachialis

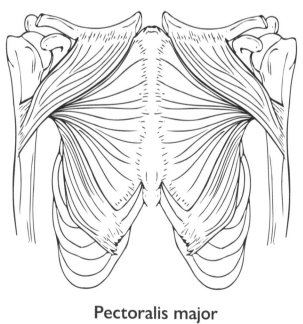

Pectoralis major

SHOULDER EXTENSORS

The shoulder extensors are a group of muscles that contract to bring the arm backwards in space. Extension of the arms is seen in poses like purvottanasana (reverse plank) and ustrasana (camel pose). The shoulder extensors are often under-used due to all of the forwards-bringing arm movements that exist in day-to-day activities. Inactive muscles weaken over time and can create imbalances in the body. In order to strengthen the shoulder extensors, yoga poses and movements that bring the arm into extension will create strength in the shoulder extensors. Some yoga poses that strengthen the extensors are purvottanasana (reverse plank), ustrasana (camel pose), and salambhasana (locust pose) with the arms back. Strengthening these muscles will begin to restore balance and mobility to the shoulder blades, which can increase the longevity and health of the shoulder joint.

SHOULDER EXTENSORS

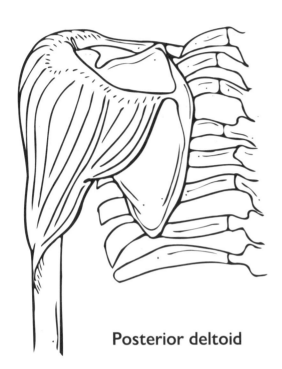

Posterior deltoid

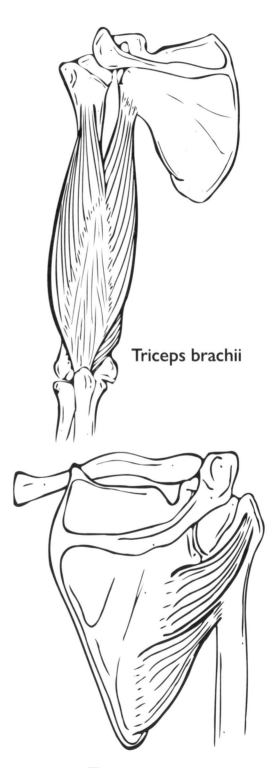

Triceps brachii

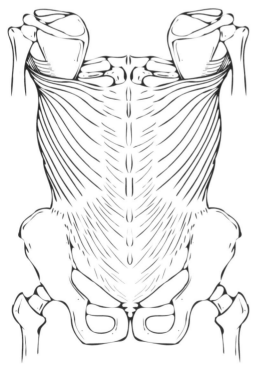

Latissimus dorsi

Teres major

SCAPULAR RETRACTION AND SCAPULAR PROTRACTION

Scapular retraction and protraction are movements that slide the shoulder blades (scapulae) in towards (retraction) or away from (protraction) the midline of the body. Retraction of the shoulder blades is often coupled with shoulder and spine extension, while protraction of the shoulder blades is often coupled with shoulder and spine flexion. Strong and balanced scapular retractor and protractor muscles help bring stability to the scapulothoracic joint (between the shoulder blades and the ribcage). A stable scapulothoracic joint will help the whole shoulder joint produce stable and healthy movements.

To activate the scapular retractors

Come into a hands and knees position with a neutral spine. Line the shoulders over the wrists and press the palms evenly into the floor. Align the hips over the knees and press the shins into the floor. Stabilize the scapulothoracic joint and begin to extend the whole spine towards the floor to come into bitilasana (cow pose). Lift the head to look up towards the ceiling. Hold this pose for 10–30 seconds with a relaxed breath. Come back into a neutral spine position.

What did you notice? Can you feel your shoulder blades retracting in towards each other? Did the movement feel stiff and weak? Or maybe strong and stable?

To activate the shoulder protractors

From a hands and knees position with a neutral spine, stabilize the scapulothoracic joint and begin to flex the whole spine, rounding it up towards the ceiling to come into marjaryasana (cat pose). Drop the head to look underneath you. Hold this position for 10–30 seconds.

What did you notice? Did you feel tight muscles between the shoulder blades lengthen and relaxing? This may indicate that your retractors are activated often.

Couple these movements 10 times and take the spine and shoulder blades through a cat and cow series.

SCAPULAR RETRACTION AND SCAPULAR PROTRACTION

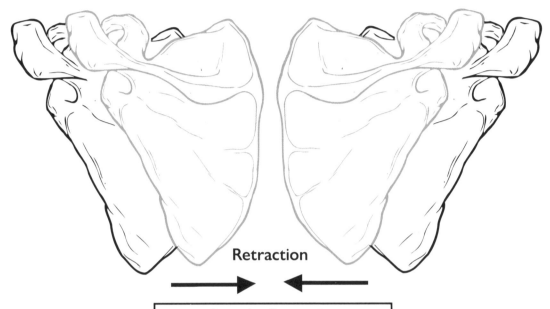

Retraction

Scapular Retraction
A movement that slides the scapula in towards the midline of the body

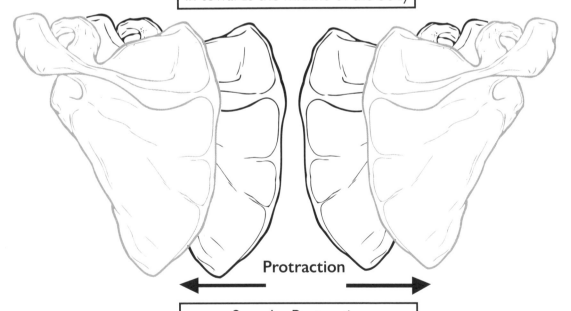

Protraction

Scapular Protraction
A movement that slides the scapula away from the midline of the body

SCAPULAR RETRACTORS

The scapular retractors are a group of muscles that contract to bring the shoulder blades in towards the midline of the body. Also referred to as scapular adductors, the muscles responsible for retracting the scapula are: the trapezius (transverse fibers), the rhomboid major, the rhomboid minor, and the serratus anterior. If the scapular retractors become weak, the shoulder joint becomes unstable and chance of injury increases during yoga poses that put the weight of the body onto the shoulder joints. Yoga poses or movements that retract the scapula will bring strength to the muscles and prepare them for more weight-bearing yoga poses. Bitilasana (cow pose) and matsyasana (fish pose) are two poses that retract the scapula and bring strength to the shoulder retractors.

SCAPULAR RETRACTORS

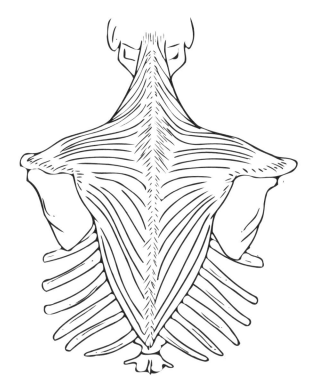

Trapezius (transverse fibers)

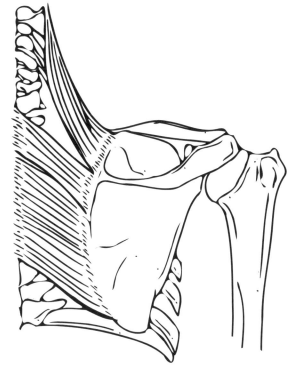

Rhomboid major and minor

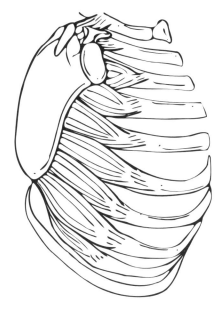

Serratus anterior

SCAPULAR PROTRACTORS

The scapular protractors, also referred to as scapular abductors, are a group of muscles that contract to slide the shoulder blades away from the midline during abduction of the arm. This provides a strong and stable foundation for the raised arm. The muscles that produce protraction are: the pectoralis minor, the pectoralis major, and the serratus anterior. If the protractors become weak, their ability to support the arm during movement decreases and the shoulder joint becomes less stable. Yoga poses or movements that abduct the arm and shoulder blades will bring strength to the muscles of protraction. Vasisthasana (side plank pose) is a pose that requires scapular protraction and will bring strength to those muscles.

SCAPULAR PROTRACTORS

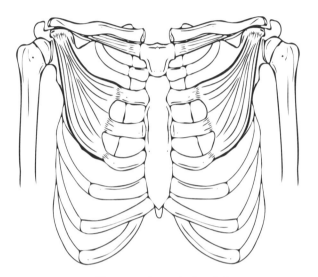

Posterior deltoid

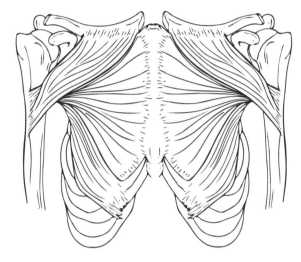

Pectoralis major

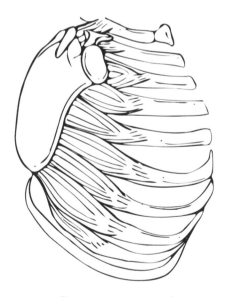

Serratus anterior

UPWARD ROTATION AND DOWNWARD ROTATION OF THE SCAPULA

Upward and downward rotations of the scapula are movements that rotate the inferior tip of the scapula away from (upward rotation) or towards (downward rotation) the midline of the body. Upward rotation of the scapulae is often coupled with shoulder abduction, while downward rotation is often coupled with shoulder adduction. Keeping the muscles of upward and downward rotation strong and balanced will help stabilize the scapulothoracic joint/shoulder joint to create stable and healthy movements.

To activate the upward rotators
Standing in mountain pose with the palms facing forwards, stabilize the scapulothoracic joint. Keep the pelvis stable and the abdominals engaged. Begin to abduct the arms out and over the head by initiating the movement from the shoulder (instead of the wrists). Hold arms overhead for 10–30 seconds.

To activate the downward rotators
Standing in mountain pose with your arms raised overhead, keep your scapulothoracic joint stable and adduct your arms back to your sides.

Couple these two movements and repeat 5–10 times.

What did you notice? Did your shoulder joint feel stable? Weak? Strong? Can you feel your shoulder blades rotating in and out as the arms move?

UPWARD ROTATION AND DOWNWARD ROTATION OF THE SCAPULA

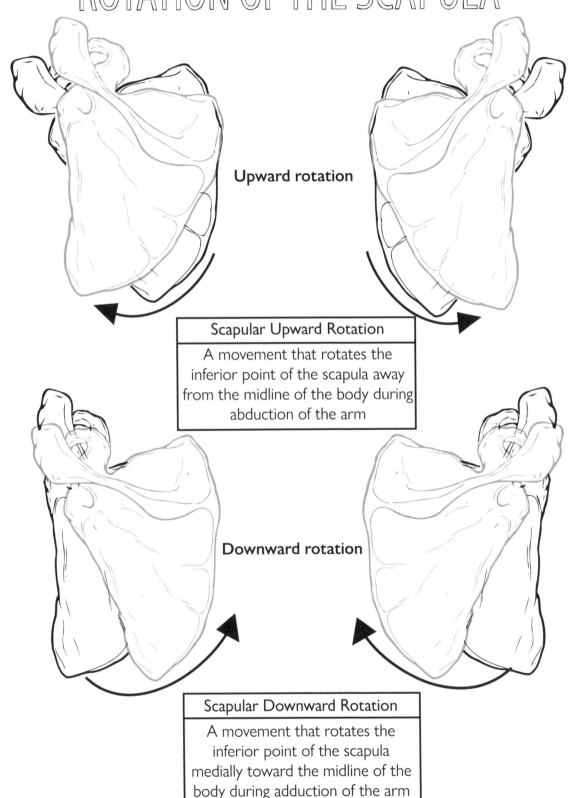

Upward rotation

Scapular Upward Rotation

A movement that rotates the inferior point of the scapula away from the midline of the body during abduction of the arm

Downward rotation

Scapular Downward Rotation

A movement that rotates the inferior point of the scapula medially toward the midline of the body during adduction of the arm

SCAPULAR UPWARD ROTATORS

The scapular upward rotators are a group of muscles that contract to rotate the inferior angle of the scapula away from the midline of the body during abduction and flexion of the arm. The muscles responsible for upward rotation of the scapula are: the trapezius and the serratus anterior. Weak upward rotators can create instability in the shoulder joint which can lead to an increased chance of injury during movement. Yoga poses or movements that bring the shoulders into upward rotation bring strength to the upward rotators. Virabhadrasana I (warrior I) strengthens the upward rotators of the scapula while the arms are brought over the head. In order to make sure the upward rotators are working efficiently, try to consciously stabilize the shoulder blades while lifting the arms in order to help the body activate and strengthen the upward rotator muscles.

SCAPULAR UPWARD ROTATORS

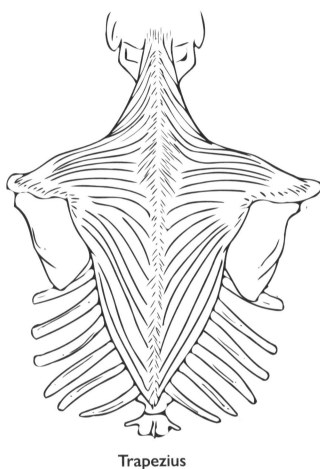

Trapezius

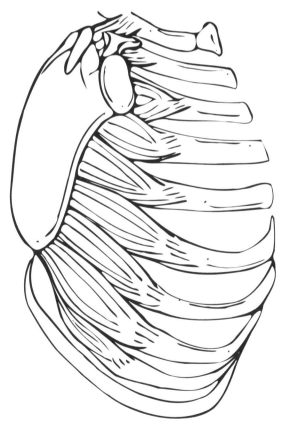

Serratus anterior

SCAPULAR DOWNWARD ROTATORS

The scapular downward rotators are a group of muscles that contract to rotate the inferior angle of the scapula inward towards the midline. This rotation of the scapula occurs when the arms are being adducted back towards the body. The muscles responsible for the downward rotation of the scapula are: the pectoralis minor, the subclavius, the pectoralis major, and the latissimus dorsi. When these muscles are weak, the shoulder joint becomes unstable during movements of adduction. Coming in and out of virabhadrasana I and II (warrior I and II) or movements that bring the arms over head and back down to the body will help strengthen the downward rotators of the scapula. In order to make sure the muscles are working efficiently, bring conscious stability to your shoulder blades as you move your arms above and below your head. This will help the downward rotators activate and will bring strength to the muscles.

SCAPULAR DOWNWARD ROTATORS

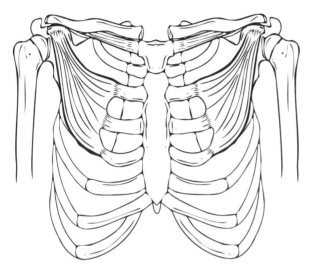

Pectoralis minor and subclavius

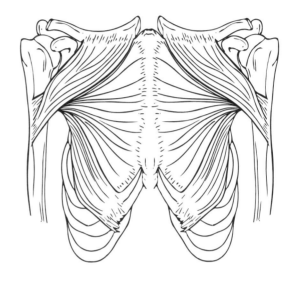

Pectoralis major

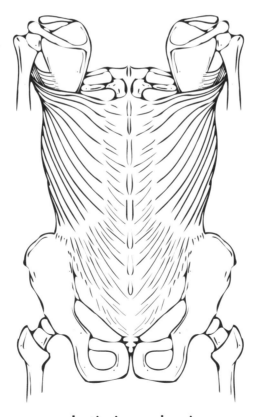

Latissimus dorsi

SCAPULAR ELEVATION AND SCAPULAR DEPRESSION

Scapular elevation and depression are movements that occur when muscles contract to raise or lower the shoulder blades (scapulae). Scapular elevation is often coupled with shoulder extension, while scapular depression is often coupled with shoulder flexion. Strong and balanced scapular elevators and depressors assist with scapulothoracic stabilization and will help bring stability and support to the whole shoulder joint as the arms move. A stable shoulder joint will create efficient and healthy movements and increase the longevity of the joint.

To activate scapular elevators

Standing in mountain pose, stabilize your shoulder at the scapulothoracic joint. Without moving the arms, try to lift the shoulder blades superiorly, sliding them up towards the head. The movement is small. Resist shrugging the shoulders up towards the ears.

To activate the scapular depressors

Standing in mountain pose, stabilize the scapulothoracic joint and raise the shoulder blades superiorly. Then, lower the shoulder blades by depressing then inferiorly towards the feet.

Couple these two movements by lifting and lowering the shoulder blades on the spine. Repeat 10–20 times.

What do you notice? Can you feel the muscles in the shoulder blades engaging to push the blades upwards and downwards? Are there any areas of tension or relief?

SCAPULAR ELEVATION AND SCAPULAR DEPRESSION

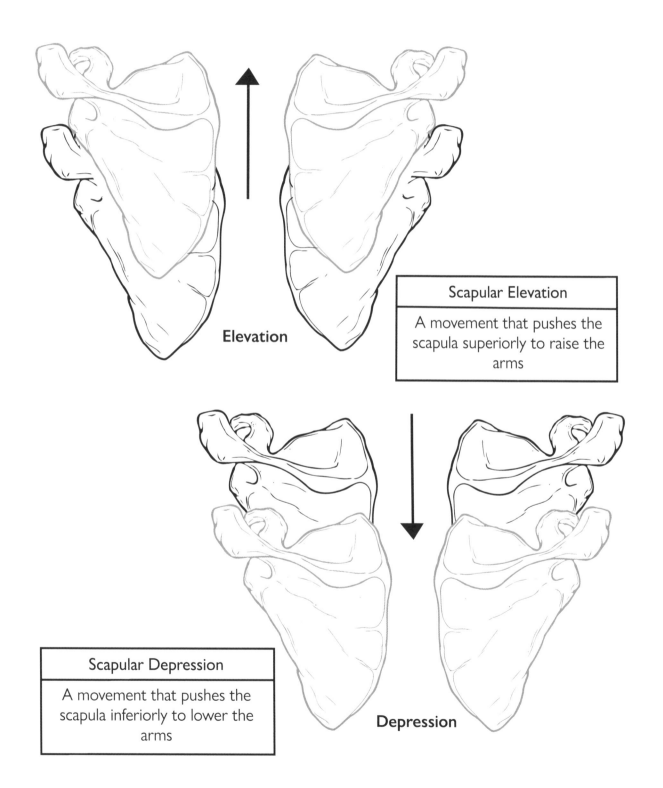

Elevation

Scapular Elevation
A movement that pushes the scapula superiorly to raise the arms

Scapular Depression
A movement that pushes the scapula inferiorly to lower the arms

Depression

SCAPULAR ELEVATORS

The scapular elevators are a group of muscles that contract to raise the shoulder blades superiorly. As the arms go from a raised position to a lowered position, the shoulder blades are elevated from depression. The muscles responsible for scapular elevation are: the trapezius (descending fibers), the rhomboid major, the rhomboid minor, and the levator scapulae. If the muscles of elevation become tight, the shoulder blades are drawn upward, creating a hunched shoulder effect. This postural behavior brings the shoulder joint out of alignment and can lead to discomfort in the shoulder joint. To lengthen the muscles of elevation, poses that require the arms to raise over the head and the shoulder blades to depress help bring length to the scapular elevators. If you feel that your scapular elevators are tight, try to actively (and gently) depress the shoulder blades as the arms are going above the head. This will help the shoulder depressors activate and signal the elevators to lengthen. If these muscles become weak, the shoulder blades become unstable during movement and this can increase the chance of injury. To strengthen the scapular elevators, yoga poses or movements that require the arms to produce adduction and the shoulder blades to elevate will bring strength to these muscles.

SCAPULAR ELEVATORS

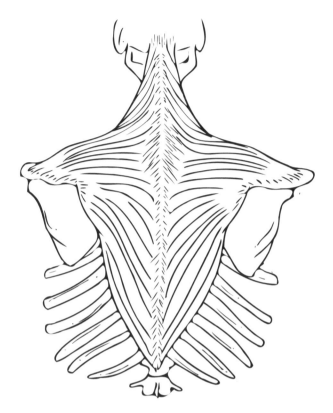

Trapezius (descending fibers)

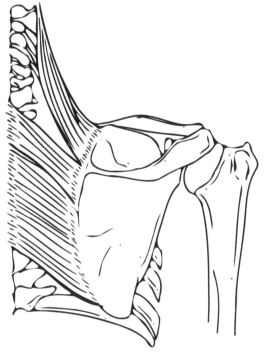

Rhomboid major and minor
with levator scapulae

SCAPULAR DEPRESSORS

The shoulder depressors are a group of muscles that contract to push the shoulder blades down the back. The shoulder blades depress as the arm raises. The muscles responsible for depression of the shoulder blades are: the pectoralis minor, the subclavius, the latissimus dorsi, and the trapezius (ascending fibers). When the shoulder depressors are tight, the shoulder joint can feel stiff and limit mobility. To lengthen the shoulder depressor muscles, yoga poses and movements that raise or elevate the shoulder blades will help loosen up the muscles of depression. If the shoulder depressors are weak, the shoulder joint may become unstable, increasing risk of injury. To strengthen the shoulder depressors, yoga poses and movements that bring the shoulder into depression will bring strength to the muscles. Yoga poses like vrksasana (tree pose) and virabhadrasana I (warrior I) require the arms to raise. This depresses the shoulder blades and begins to strengthen the muscles of depression.

SCAPULAR DEPRESSORS

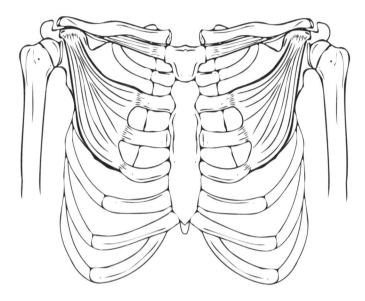

Pectoralis minor and subclavius

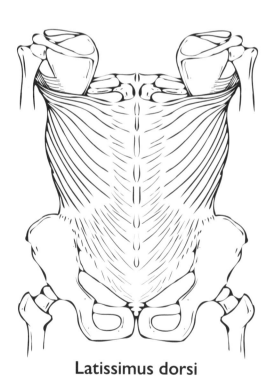

Latissimus dorsi

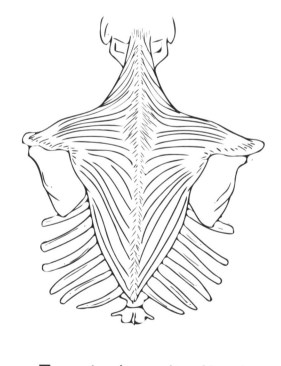

Trapezius (ascending fibers)

ANTERIOR DELTOID

The deltoid muscle is located on the lateral ball of the shoulder. It covers the glenohumeral joint and is responsible for a wide range of movements. Since the variety of movements varies, the deltoid can be broken down into three sections: the anterior deltoid, the middle deltoid, and the posterior deltoid. The deltoid produces different movements, which means the muscle works antagonistically against itself.

The anterior deltoid is the anterior part of the deltoid muscle. The anterior deltoid originates on the lateral one third of the clavicle bone and runs across the anterior shoulder joint to insert into the deltoid tuberosity of the humerus bone. When the fibers contract, the anterior deltoid is responsible for flexing and internally rotating the humerus bone at the glenohumeral joint. Overly tight anterior deltoid muscles shorten and can limit the muscle's ability to lengthen during shoulder extension. To lengthen these muscles, gently practicing yoga poses or movements that bring the shoulders into extension will work to bring length to the anterior deltoids. If the anterior deltoids become weak due to inactivity, the shoulder joint will become less stable in poses like adho mukha vrksasana (handstand) and chaturanga dandasana (four-limbed staff pose). This can increase the chances of injury to the shoulder joint. To strengthen the anterior deltoids, practicing poses or movements that gradually put weight onto the muscles during flexion will begin to strengthen the muscles. Poses like adho mukha svanasana (downward facing dog) or ardha pincha mayurasana (dolphin pose) are two poses that put weight onto the anterior deltoids and will strengthen the shoulder joint and prepare the muscles for more weight-bearing poses. For example, when the anterior deltoids contract to flex the arm forwards, the posterior deltoids lengthen, and vise versa.

ANTERIOR DELTOID

Action: Flexion and internal rotation of the arm at the shoulder joint

Origin: Lateral one third of clavicle

Insertion: Deltoid tuberosity of humerus

Agonists: *Flexion:* biceps brachii, coracobrachialis, pectoralis major

Antagonists: *Flexion:* posterior deltoid, triceps brachii, latissimus dorsi, pectoralis major, teres major

Poses: *Contracts:* adho mukha svanasana, adho mukha vrksasana, bitilasana. *Lengthens:* purvottanasana

Anterior deltoid

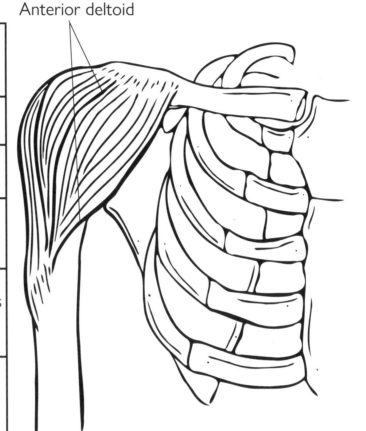

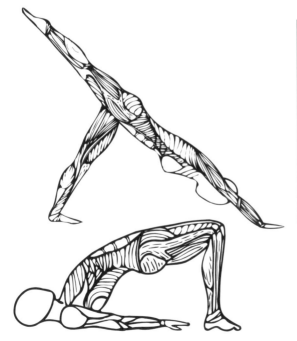

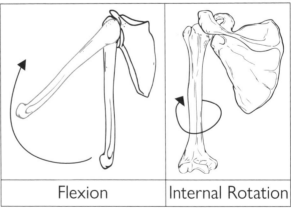

| Flexion | Internal Rotation |

Posterior view

MIDDLE DELTOID

The middle deltoids are part of the deltoid muscles. Originating on the acromion of the scapula, the middle deltoids extend down towards the humerus bone and insert onto the deltoid tuberosity of the humerus bone. When the fibers of the middle deltoids contract, they pull the arms into abduction. If the middle deltoids become weak, their ability to hold weight during abduction decreases and chance of injury to the shoulder joint increases during movements. Poses or movements that bring the arm into abduction will increase the strength of the middle deltoids. Vasisthasana (side plank pose) abducts the arms and puts weight onto the shoulder joint, giving opportunity for the middle deltoids to gain strength. If vasisthasana puts too much weight onto the shoulder joint and pain or discomfort occurs, a variation of vasisthasana with the knee pressing into the ground will help take some of the weight off the shoulders. This allows the middle deltoids to slowly build strength with a lower weight. If the muscles are feeling tight, yoga poses or movements that bring the arms into adduction will lengthen the fibers of the middle deltoid.

MIDDLE DELTOID

Action: Abduction of the arm at the shoulder joint

Origin: Acromion of the scapula

Insertion: Deltoid tuberosity of the humerus

Agonists: Anterior deltoid, posterior deltoid

Antagonists: Latissimus dorsi, pectoralis major, teres major, triceps brachii

Poses: *Contracts:* vasisthasana, virabhadrasana II. *Lengthens:* garudasana (poses with adduction)

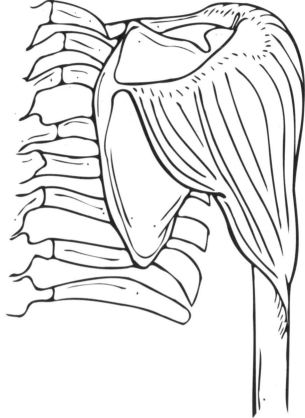

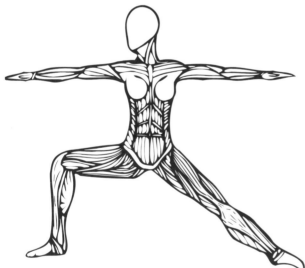

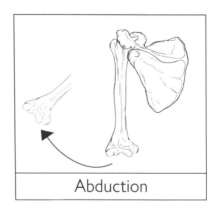

Abduction

Posterior view

POSTERIOR DELTOID

The posterior deltoid is part of the deltoid muscle located on the posterior side of the shoulder. It originates on the spine of the scapula and joins with the rest of the deltoid to insert into the deltoid tuberosity of the humerus bone. The fibers of the posterior deltoids contract to produce extension and external rotation of the shoulder joint. In a forwards-facing world, the posterior deltoids can often be overlooked. With so many opportunities for forwards-flexing shoulder movements, extension of the shoulder joint is easy to neglect. A lack of extension can cause the posterior deltoids to become weak or inactive. In order to bring strength to the muscles, yoga poses or movements that bring the arm into extension will begin to activate and strengthen the posterior deltoids. Purvottanasana (upward plank pose) or a variation of purvottanasana, with the knees bent at a 90-degree angle, are two ways to bring strength to the posterior deltoids. Another characteristic to note about the deltoids is that when the posterior deltoids contract to extend or externally rotate the arm, the anterior deltoids lengthen.

POSTERIOR DELTOID

Action: Extension and external rotation of the arm at the shoulder joint

Origin: Scapular spine of the shoulder blade

Insertion: Deltoid tuberosity of the humerus

Agonists: *Extension:* triceps brachii (LH), latissimus dorsi, pectoralis major, teres major. *External rotation:* infraspinatus, teres major

Antagonists: *Extension:* anterior deltoid, biceps brachii, coracobrachialis, pectoralis major. *External rotation:* anterior deltoid, teres major, latissimus dorsi, pectoralis major, subscapularis

Poses: *Contracts:* purvottanasana. *Lengthens:* kumbhakasana

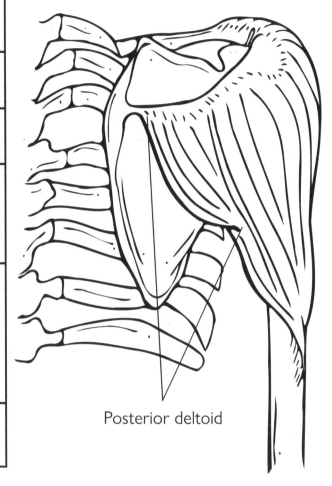

Posterior deltoid

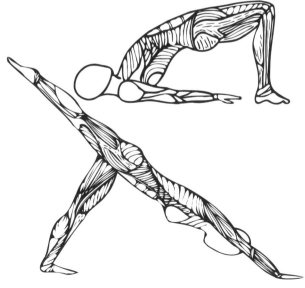

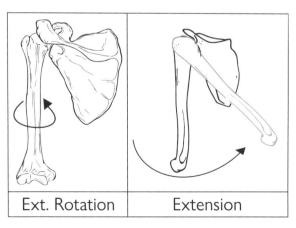

Ext. Rotation | Extension

Posterior view

BICEPS BRACHII

The biceps brachii muscle is a multi-headed muscle with two origin sites. The muscle is broken down into two heads: the long head (LH) and the short head (SH). The long head originates on the supraglenoid tubercle of the scapula, while the short head originates on the coracoid process of the scapula. The muscle extends down, crosses over the elbow joint, and inserts onto the radial tuberosity of the radius bone. Since the biceps brachii crosses over two joints, the shoulder joint and the elbow joint, it produces multiple movements. When contracted, the muscle produces flexion and supination of the forearm, and assists with flexion, abduction, and internal rotation of the humerus at the shoulder joint. The biceps brachii also plays a role in providing shoulder stabilization.

BICEPS BRACHII

Action: Flexion and supination at elbow joint. Flexion and stabilization of shoulder joint, abduction and internal rotation of humerus

Origin: Supraglenoid tubercle of scapula (LH). Coracoid process of scapula (SH)

Insertion: Radial tuberosity

Agonists: *Flexion of elbow joint:* brachialis, brachioradialis. *Flexion of arm at shoulder:* deltoid anterior, coracobrachialis, pectoralis major. *Supination:* supinator

Antagonists: *Flexion of elbow joint:* triceps brachii, anconeus. *Flexion of arm at shoulder:* deltoid posterior, triceps brachii (LH), latissimus dorsi, pectoralis major, teres major. *Supination:* pronator teres, pronator quadratus

Poses: *Contracts:* bakasana, chaturanga dandasana, salamba bhujangasana. *Lengthens:* kumbhakasana, marjaryasana, bitilasana, virabhadrasana I and II

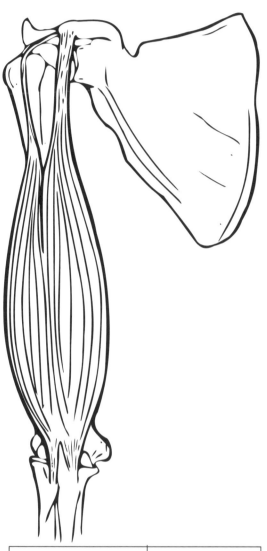

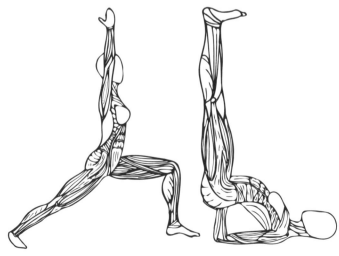

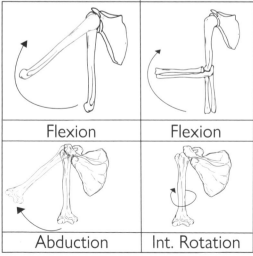

Flexion	Flexion
Abduction	Int. Rotation

Posterior view

CORACOBRACHIALIS

The coracobrachialis is located on the anterior superior medial portion of the humerus bone. It shares an origination site on the coracoid process of the scapula with the biceps brachii (SH) and the pectoralis minor. It extends down to insert onto the crest of the lesser tuberosity of the humerus bone. When contracted, the coracobrachialis assists with flexion, adduction, and internal rotation of the humerus bone at the shoulder joint.

CORACOBRACHIALIS

Action: Flexion, adduction, internal rotation of humerus at shoulder joint

Origin: Coracoid process of scapula

Insertion: Crest of lesser tuberosity of humerus

Agonists: *Flexion:* deltoid anterior, biceps brachii, pectoralis major. *Adduction:* latissimus dorsi, teres major, pectoralis major, triceps brachii (LH)

Antagonists: *Flexion:* deltoid posterior, triceps brachii (LH), latissimus dorsi, pectoralis major, teres major. *Adduction:* middle deltoid, supraspinatus

Poses: *Contracts:* kumbhakasana. *Lengthens:* purvottanasana, virabhadrasana I

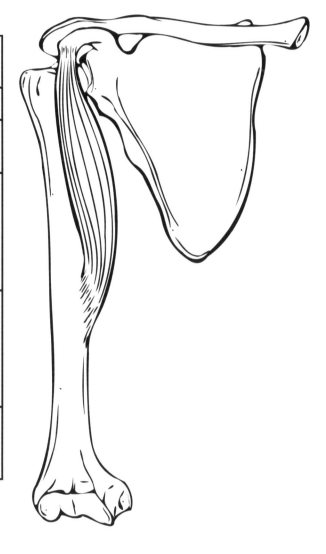

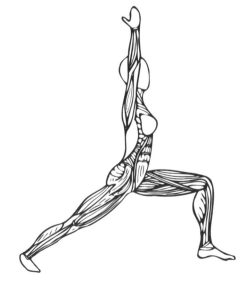

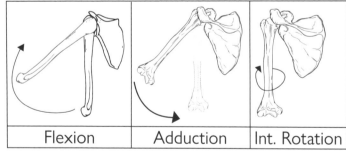

| Flexion | Adduction | Int. Rotation |

Posterior view

INFRASPINATUS

The infraspinatus is one of the four muscles that make up the Rotators Cuff group. It originates on the infraspinous fossa located on the posterior side of the scapula. The muscle runs across the glenohumeral joint and attaches to the greater tuberosity of the humerus bone. When the fibers contract, the infraspinatus pulls the humerus into external rotation. The infraspinatus can become weak when postural habits start to favor internal rotation. Since the infraspinatus is also a shoulder stabilizer, when it becomes weak shoulder stability decreases. With a weak or overly tight infraspinatus, the chances of tearing the tendon or muscle increase during movement. Yoga poses or movements that bring the arms into external rotation will bring strength and stability to the infraspinatus. Virabhadrasana II (warrior II) with the palms facing towards the sky and adho mukha svanasana (downward facing dog) are two poses that bring the arms into external rotation and will bring strength to the infraspinatus. A strong and stable shoulder joint increases the joint's longevity by decreasing the chances of injury.

INFRASPINATUS

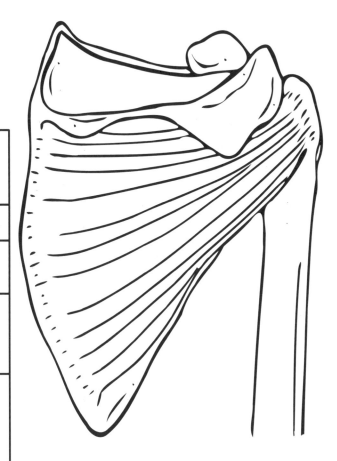

Action: External rotation of arm at shoulder joint, stabilization of shoulder joint

Origin: Infraspinous fossa of scapula

Insertion: Greater tuberosity of humerus

Agonists: Posterior deltoid, supraspinatus, teres major, teres minor, subscapularis

Antagonists: Pectoralis major, subscapularis, latissimus dorsi, teres major, coracobrachialis, anterior deltoid

Poses: *Contracts:* adho mukha svanasana. *Lengthens:* gomukhasana

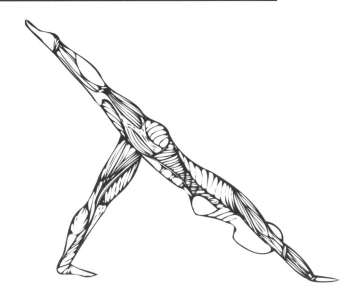

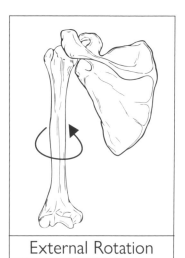

External Rotation

Posterior view

LATISSIMUS DORSI

The latissimus dorsi is a large superficial muscle that spans from the middle to low back. It can be broken up into four sections based on origin sites: the vertebral part (VP), the scapular part (SP), the costal part (CP), and the iliac part (IP). The vertebral part originates on the spinous processes of T7–T12 vertebrae and the thoracolumbar fascia. The scapular part originates on the inferior angle of the scapula. The costal part originates on ribs 9–12. And the iliac part originates on the iliac crest. The muscle spans up towards the superior portion of the humerus bone and inserts onto the lesser tuberosity of the humerus. When the different parts of the latissimus dorsi contract, the arms adduct, extend, and internally rotate at the shoulder joint. Practicing salabhasana (locust pose) with hands clasped can bring strength to the latissimus dorsi because it brings the arms into extension, internal rotation, and adduction, allowing for each part of the latissimus dorsi to simultaneously contract.

LATISSIMUS DORSI

Action: Adduction, extension, and internal rotation of the arm at the shoulder joint

Origin: Spinous process of T7–T12 vertebrae, thoracolumbar fascia (VP). Inferior angle of scapula (SP). Ribs 9th–12th (CP). Iliac crest (IP)

Insertion: Lesser tuberosity of humerus

Agonists: *Adduction:* pectoralis major, teres major, triceps brachii (LH). *Extension:* deltoid posterior, triceps brachii (LH), pectoralis major. *Internal rotation:* subscapularis, deltoid anterior, pectoralis major

Antagonists: *Adduction:* deltoid middle, supraspinatus. *Extension:* deltoid anterior, biceps brachii, coracobrachialis, pectoralis major. *Internal rotation:* infraspinatus, teres minor, deltoid posterior

Poses: *Contracts:* gomukhasana, urdhva dhanurasana, purvottanasana. *Lengthens:* balasana, utthita parsvakonasana, adho mukha svanasana

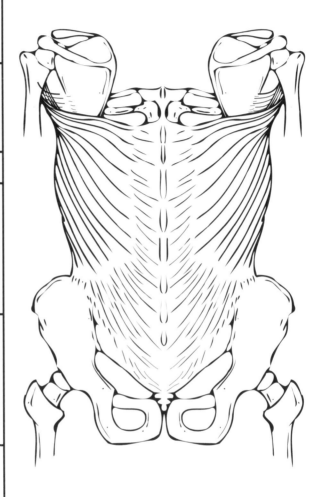

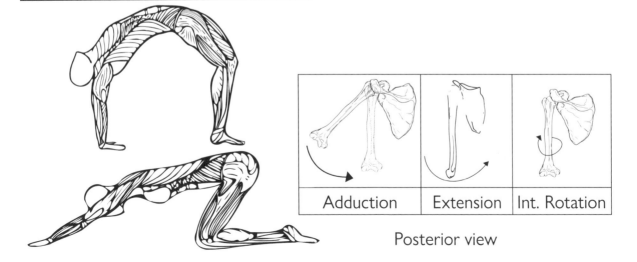

| Adduction | Extension | Int. Rotation |

Posterior view

LEVATOR SCAPULAE

The levator scapulae are muscles with a name of the function they produce. The latin word "levare" means "to lift," and the levator scapulae are responsible for lifting, or elevating, the scapula. The levator scapulae are small muscles that originate on the transverse processes of C1–C4 vertebrae and insert onto the superior angle of the scapula. When the muscles become tight from over-use, the posture of the shoulders shrug towards the ears. To lengthen the levator scapulae, yoga poses or movements that depress the shoulder blades work to elongate the muscles. As the shoulder blades depress, the muscles of shoulder depression strengthen and start to bring the shoulders back into balance.

LEVATOR SCAPULAE

Action: Elevation of scapula, downward rotation
Origin: Transverse process of C1–C4
Insertion: Superior angle of scapula
Agonists: Trapezius upper fibers
Antagonists: Trapezius lower fibers, serratus anterior, pectoralis major
Poses: *Contracts:* shoulder shrug, salabhasana, ustrasana. *Lengthens:* depression of shoulder blades, halasana

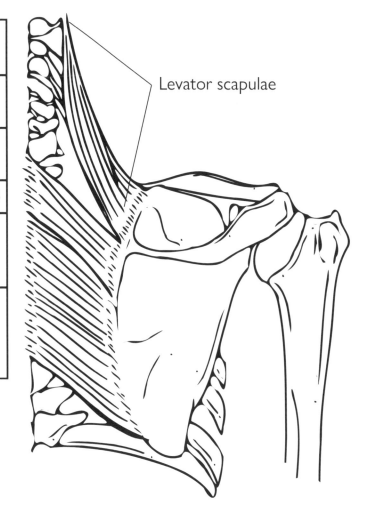

Levator scapulae

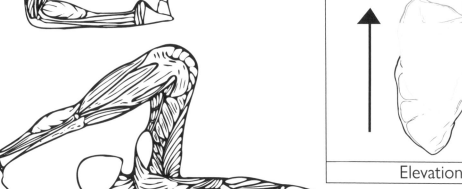

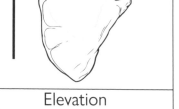

Elevation

Posterior view

PECTORALIS MAJOR

The pectoralis major is located on the anterior superior portion of the ribcage. It is split into three sections based on the origins: the clavicular part (CP), the sternocostal part (SP), and the abdominal part (AP). The clavicular part originates on the anterior surface of the clavicle bone. The sternocostal part originates on the sternum and costal cartilages of ribs 1–6. And the abdominal part originates on the rectus sheath of the transversus abdominis and internal and external oblique fibers. The fibers of each section travel towards the armpit and insert onto the crest of the greater tuberosity on the humerus bone. When the fibers contract, they produce adduction, internal rotation, and flexion of the shoulder joint. When the shoulder is fixed, the costal part and the sternal part also assist with respiration. To strengthen the pectoralis major, yoga poses and movements that produce adduction, internal rotation, and flexion of the arm will work to contract the pectoralis major. Chaturanga dandasana (four-limbed staff pose) and marjaryasana (cat pose) are two yoga poses that bring the muscles into contraction. To lengthen the muscles, poses or movements that bring the arms into abduction, extension, or external rotation will begin to elongate the muscles. Dhanurasana (bow pose) and urdhva dhanurasana (wheel pose) require the pectoralis major to lengthen. Over-tightness of the muscles will limit the depth and ability of the muscles to enter lengthening poses. Be cautious of any pain or discomfort that arises when working to lengthen the pectoralis major muscles.

PECTORALIS MAJOR

Action: Adduction, internal rotation, and flexion of shoulder joint. Respiration assistance when shoulder is in a fixed position (CP, SP)

Origin: Anterior surface of clavicle (CP). Sternum, costal cartilages 1–6 (SP). Rectus sheath (AP)

Insertion: Crest of greater tuberosity of humerus

Agonists: *Adduction:* latissimus dorsi, teres major, pectoralis major (SP), triceps brachii (LH). *Internal rotation:* latissimus dorsi, subscapularis, anterior deltoid, pectoralis major (SP), triceps brachii (LH). *Flexion:* anterior deltoid, biceps brachii, coracobrachialis

Antagonists: *Adduction:* middle deltoid supraspinatus. *Internal rotation:* infraspinatus, teres minor, posterior deltoid. *Flexion:* posterior deltoid, triceps brachii (LH), latissimus dorsi, pectoralis major (SP), teres major

Poses: *Contracts:* marjaryasana, adho mukha svanasana, chaturanga dandasana. *Lengthens:* dhanurasana, urdhva dhanurasana, virabhadrasana II

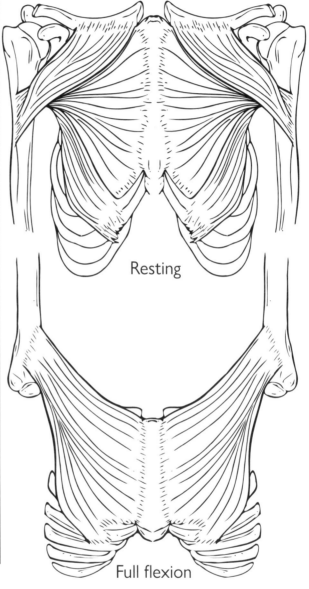

Resting

Full flexion

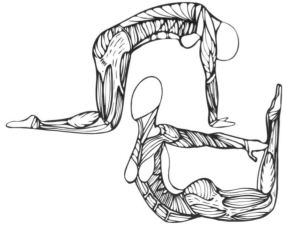

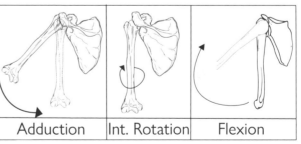

| Adduction | Int. Rotation | Flexion |

Posterior view

PECTORALIS MINOR

The pectoralis minor lies deep to the pectoralis major. It originates from the third to fifth ribs and runs up to insert onto the coracoid process of the scapula. When the fibers of the pectoralis minor contract, the shoulder blades protract and downwardly rotate. If the muscles become overly tight, they contribute to rounding the shoulders while sitting. To lengthen the pectoralis minor muscles, poses that retract the scapula (towards the midline) or bring the scapula into upward rotation will work to elongate the muscles.

PECTORALIS MINOR

Action: Protraction and downward rotation of scapula. Assists in respiration

Origin: 3rd–5th ribs

Insertion: Coracoid process

Agonists: *Protraction:* serratus anterior. *Downward rotation:* levator scapulae, serratus anterior, rhomboid major, rhomboid minor, trapezius

Antagonists: *Protraction:* trapezius, rhomboid major, rhomboid minor. *Downward rotation:* trapezius, serratus anterior

Poses: *Contracts:* marjaryasana. *Lengthens:* ustrasana, urdhva dhanurasana, matsyasana

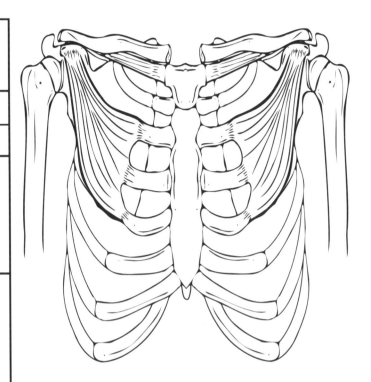

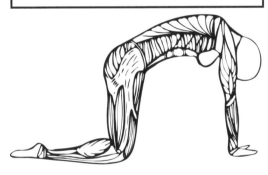

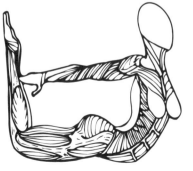

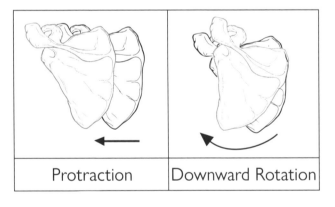

Protraction | Downward Rotation

Posterior view

RHOMBOID MAJOR

The rhomboid major is located in between the medial border of the scapula and the midline of the body. It lies superior to the rhomboid minor. Originating on the spinous process of the T1–T4 vertebrae, the rhomboid major extends towards the scapula to insert onto the medial border of the scapula. When the fibers contract, they pull the scapula in towards the midline, retracting the scapula. To lengthen the rhomboid major, yoga poses and movements that protract the scapula will begin to elongate the muscles. Marjaryasana (cat pose) requires the shoulder blades to protract and the rhomboid major to lengthen. To bring strength to the rhomboid major, yoga poses that require the shoulder blades to retract will work to contract the muscles. Bitilasana (cow pose) requires the shoulder blades to retract and will work to bring strength to the muscles.

RHOMBOID MAJOR

Action: Retraction of scapula and stabilization of shoulder blade

Origin: Spinous process of T1–T4 vertebrae

Insertion: Medial border of scapula

Agonists: Trapezius, rhomboid minor

Antagonists: Serratus anterior, pectoralis major, trapezius

Poses: *Contracts:* bitilasana, urdhva dhanurasana. *Lengthens:* setu bhanda sarvangasana, marjaryasana

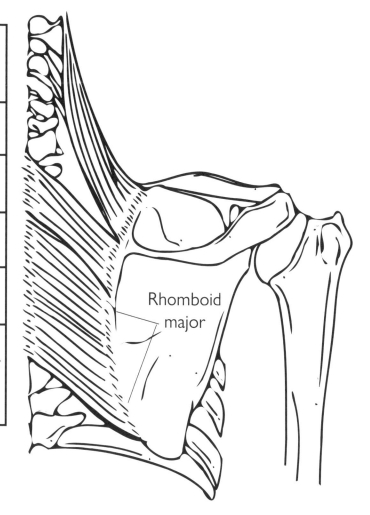

Rhomboid major

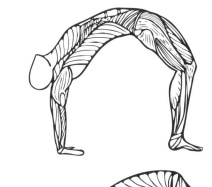

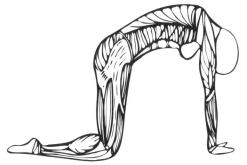

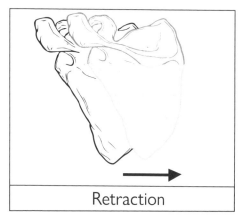

Retraction

Posterior view

RHOMBOID MINOR

The rhomboid minor lies superiorly to the rhomboid major and inferiorly to the levator scapulae. It originates on the spinous process of the C6–C7 vertebrae and inserts onto the medial border of the scapula. When the fibers of the rhomboid minor contract, the shoulder blades retract. Yoga poses or movements that bring the shoulders into protraction bring length to the rhomboid minor muscles.

RHOMBOID MINOR

Action: Retraction of shoulder blades, stabilization of shoulder joint
Origin: Spinous process C6–C7
Insertion: Medial border of scapula
Agonists: Trapezius, rhomboid major, levator scapulae, serratus anterior, rhomboid major
Antagonists: Serratus anterior upper fibers, pectoralis major
Poses: *Contracts:* urdhva dhanurasana. *Lengthens:* marjaryasana

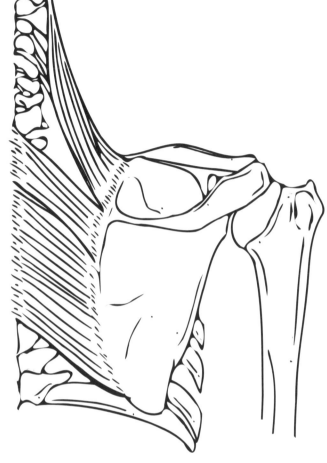

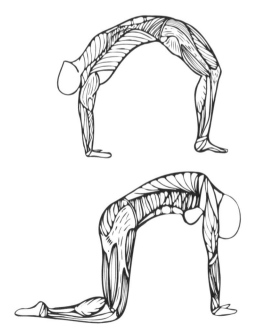

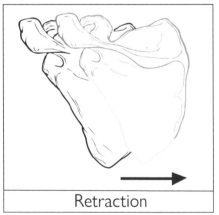

Retraction

Posterior view

SERRATUS ANTERIOR

The serratus anterior is a multi-segmented muscle located on the medial posterior side of the ribcage. Originating on ribs 1–9, the segments of the serratus anterior extend back to insert onto the medial border of the scapula. Since the segments spread and fan out, the angle of the fibers on each segment allow for the muscle to produce opposing movements. When the fibers contract, they pull the scapula into upward rotation, downward rotation, protraction, and depression. The serratus anterior also assists in abduction of the shoulder joint and works to stabilize the scapulothoracic joint formed between the scapula and the ribcage. In yoga, the serratus anterior plays an important role in stabilizing the torso in arm balances and inverted poses.

SERRATUS ANTERIOR

Action: Upward rotation, downward rotation, protraction and depression of scapula. Shoulder blade stabilization to ribcage. Abduction of shoulder joint

Origin: 1st–9th ribs

Insertion: Medial border of scapula

Agonists: *Upward rotation:* trapezius. *Downward rotation:* levator scapulae, rhomboid major, rhomboid minor, trapezius, serratus anterior (IP). *Protraction:* pectoralis major. *Depression:* pectoralis minor, trapezius

Antagonists: *Upward rotation:* levator scapulae, serratus anterior (SP). Rhomboid major, rhomboid minor, pectoralis minor. *Downward rotation:* trapezius, serratus anterior (IP). *Protraction:* trapezius, rhomboid major, rhomboid minor. *Depression:* trapezius, levator scapulae

Poses: *Contracts:* dandasana, chaturanga (dandasana), adho mukha vrksasana, bakasana. *Lengthens:* parighasana, viparita virabhadrasana, parsva urdhva hastasana

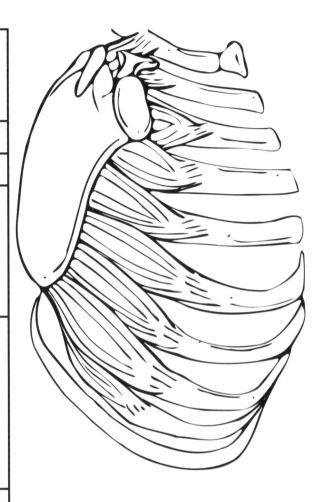

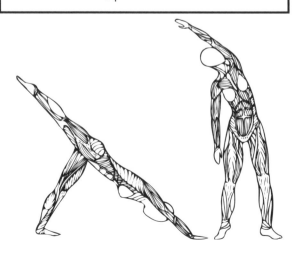

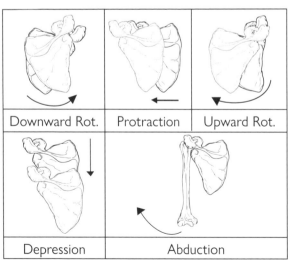

Downward Rot.	Protraction	Upward Rot.
Depression	Abduction	

Posterior view

SUBSCAPULARIS

The subscapularis is one of the four muscles that make up the Rotators Cuff. It originates in the subscapular fossa on the anterior side of the scapula. It crosses over the glenohumeral joint and inserts onto the lesser tuberosity of the humerus bone. When the fibers of the subscapularis contract, they pull the humerus bone into internal rotation. Due to postural behaviors, the subscapularis can become tight from prolonged internal rotation of the arms. In order to lengthen the subscapularis, poses that require external rotation will work to elongate the fibers of the muscle. This will also bring strength to the external rotators. As the external rotators become stronger, the posture of the shoulders will begin to balance.

SUBSCAPULARIS

Action: Internal rotation, adduction of arm
Origin: Subscapular fossa of scapula
Insertion: Lesser tuberosity of humerus
Agonists: Teres major, latissimus dorsi, pectoralis major
Antagonists: Infraspinatus, teres minor
Poses: *Contracts:* setu bandhasana, gomukhasana, anjali mudra. *Lengthens:* adho mukha svanasana

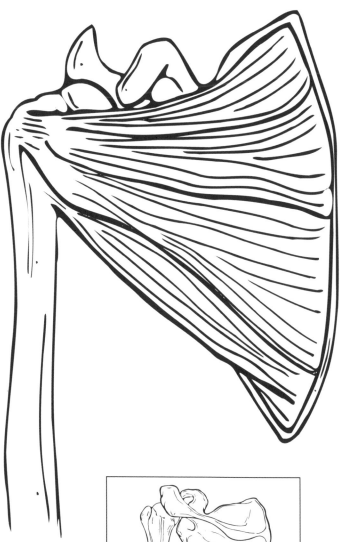

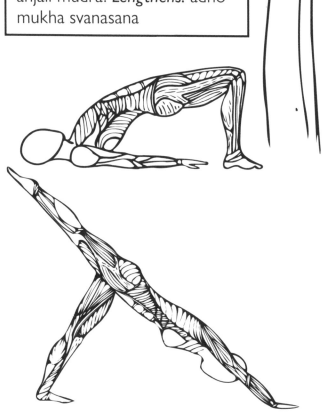

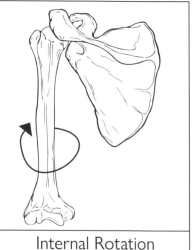

Internal Rotation

Posterior view

SUPRASPINATUS

The supraspinatus is one of the four muscles that make up the Rotators Cuff. It is a small muscle that originates on the superior posterior portion of the scapula. Originating on the supraspinous fossa, the supraspinatus extends across the superior portion of the glenohumeral joint and inserts onto the greater tuberosity of the humerus bone. When the fibers contract, the supraspinatus assists in abduction of the humerus bone.

SUPRASPINATUS

Action: Abduction of arm at shoulder joint, stabilizes humerus

Origin: Supraspinous fossa of scapula

Insertion: Greater tuberosity of humerus

Agonists: Deltoid, infraspinatus, teres major, teres minor, subscapularis

Antagonists: Pectoralis major, latissimus dorsi, teres major, pectoralis minor, subclavius, serratus anterior, trapezius, rhomboid major, rhomboid minor, levator scapulae

Poses: *Contracts:* virabhadrasana II. *Lengthens:* garudasana, adho mukha vrksasana

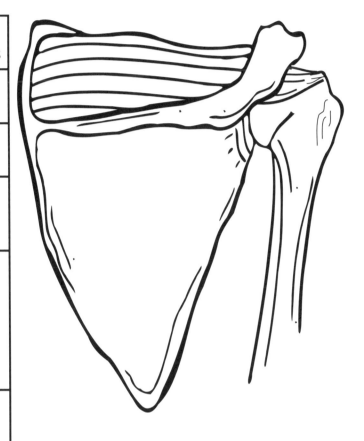

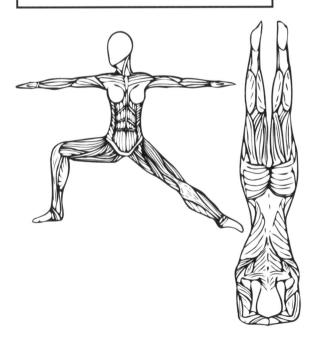

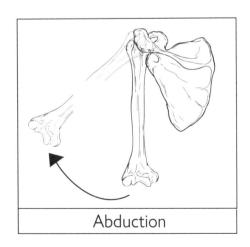

Abduction

Posterior view

TERES MAJOR

The teres major is a small muscle that originates on the inferior angle of the scapula. The muscle fibers run towards the lateral body and insert onto the lesser tuberosity of the anterior humerus bone. When contracted, the teres major is responsible for internally rotating, adducting, and extending the humerus bone. It also plays a role in providing stability to the shoulder joint during inverted yoga poses.

TERES MAJOR

Action: Internal rotation, adduction, and extension of humerus. Stabilizes shoulder joint

Origin: Inferior angle of scapula

Insertion: Lesser tuberosity of humerus

Agonists: *Internal rotation:* subscapularis, deltoid, latissimus dorsi, pectoralis major. *Adduction:* latissimus dorsi, pectoralis major, triceps brachii. *Extension:* deltoid, triceps brachii, latissimus dorsi, pectoralis major

Antagonists: *Internal rotation:* infraspinatus, teres minor, deltoid. *Adduction:* deltoid, supraspinatus. *Extension:* deltoid, biceps brachii, coracobrachialis, pectoralis major

Poses: *Contracts:* garudasana. *Lengthens:* adho mukha svanasana

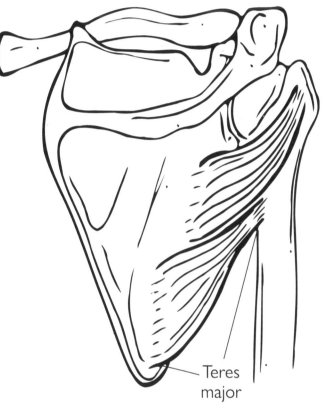

Teres major

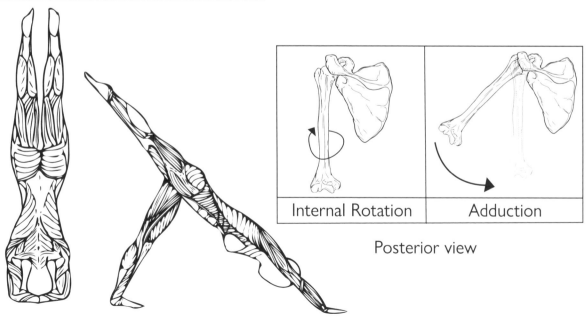

Internal Rotation | Adduction

Posterior view

TERES MINOR

The teres minor is one of the four muscles that make up the Rotators Cuff. It is located on the posterior lateral scapula and sits superiorly to the teres major. Originating on the lateral border of the scapula, the teres minor crosses over the glenohumeral joint and shares an insertion point with the infraspinatus on the greater tuberosity of the humerus bone. When the fibers of the muscle contract, the teres minor assists with external rotation of the humerus bone. The teres minor also works to stabilize the shoulder joint during movement.

TERES MINOR

Action: External rotation and weak adduction of humerus

Origin: Lateral border of scapula

Insertion: Greater tuberosity of humerus

Agonists: *External rotation:* infraspinatus, deltoid

Antagonists: *External rotation:* deltoid, subscapularis, pectoralis major, teres major, latissimus dorsi

Poses: *Contracts:* adho mukha svanasana. *Lengthens:* garudasana, adho mukha vrksasana

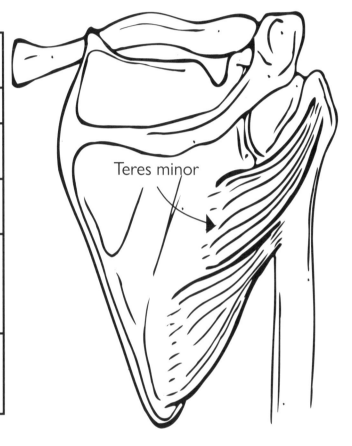

Teres minor

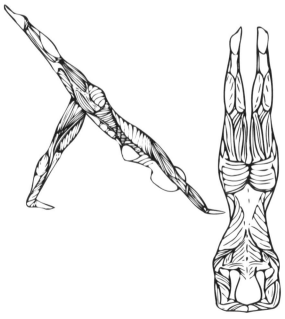

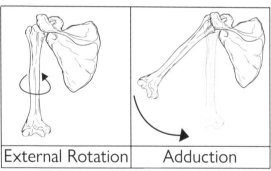

| External Rotation | Adduction |

Posterior view

TRAPEZIUS

The trapezius is a kite-shaped muscle that extends from the occipital protuberance of the skull, to the lateral spine of the scapula, and down to the last thoracic vertebrae. The trapezius can be broken up into three parts based on the run of the muscle fibers: the descending part (DP), the transverse part (TP), and the ascending part (AP). The descending part originates on the occipital protuberance of the skull and the spinous process of C1–C7 vertebrae. The fibers descend down to insert onto the lateral third of the clavicle bone. The transverse part originates on the aponeurosis (fibrous sheath) near the T1–T4 spinous process and inserts onto the acromion of the scapula. The ascending part originates on the spinous process of T5–T12. The fibers ascend upwards to insert onto the spine of the scapula. When the muscle fibers of the trapezius contract, the scapula elevates (DP), retracts (TP), and depresses (TP, AP). The trapezius is also responsible for abducting the humerus bone and stabilizing the scapulothoracic joint.

When the fibers of the trapezius become tight, they can pull on the neck and cause tension headaches as well as attribute to poor and rounded posture. Since the different parts of the trapezius control different movements of the scapula, lengthening the muscle depends on the area of tightness. If the superior shoulders and neck feel tight, movements that depress the scapula will lengthen the descending part of the trapezius. If the shoulder blades feel tight and squeezed together, movements that protract the scapula will bring length to the transverse part and ascending part. And since the trapezius plays a role in arm abduction, yoga poses and movements that bring the arm into adduction will also bring length to the trapezius.

TRAPEZIUS

Action: Elevation (DP), retraction (TP), and depression of scapula (TP, AP). Abduction of humerus at shoulder joint. Stabilization of scapula and thorax

Origin: Occipital bone and spinous process C1–C7 (DP), aponeurosis spinous process T1–T4 (TP), spinous process of T5–T12 (AP)

Insertion: Lateral one third of clavicle (DP), acromion (TP), scapular spine (AP)

Agonists: Serratus anterior lower fibers, trapezius (DP), rhomboid major, rhomboid minor, serratus anterior

Antagonists: Levator scapulae, serratus anterior (DP), rhomboid major and minor, pectoralis minor (DP), serratus anterior, pectoralis minor (TP), trapezius upper fibers, levator scapulae (AP)

Poses: *Contracts:* adho mukha vrksasana, bakasana. *Lengthens:* balasana, garudasana

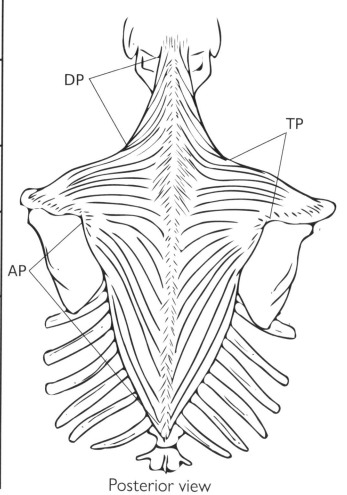

DP
TP
AP

Posterior view

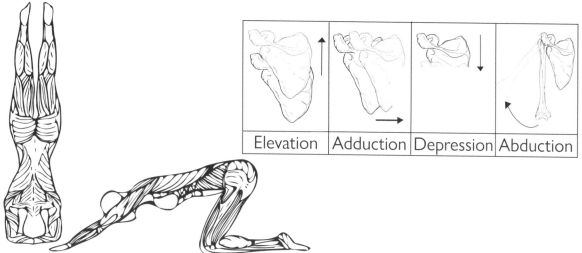

| Elevation | Adduction | Depression | Abduction |

TRICEPS BRACHII

The triceps brachii is a long multi-headed muscle that extends along the posterior humerus bone. The triceps brachii consists of three heads: the long head (LH), the short head (SH), and the lateral head (LatH). The long head originates on the infraglenoid tubercle of the scapula. The short head and lateral head originate on the posterior humerus bone. They all come together to cross over the elbow joint to insert onto the olecranon of the ulna bone. When the fibers of the full triceps brachii contract, they shorten and pull the elbow into extension. Since the long head attaches to the posterior scapula, when the long head fibers contract they assist with extension and adduction of the shoulder joint. To lengthen tight tricep muscles, yoga poses or movements that bring the elbow into flexion and the shoulder into flexion or abduction will work to elongate the tricep muscles.

TRICEPS BRACHII

Action: Extension of elbow joint. Extension and adduction of shoulder joint (LH)

Origin: Infraglenoid tubercle of scapula (LH). Posterior superior humerus (SH). Posterior superior humerus (LatH)

Insertion: Olecranon of ulna

Agonists: *Shoulder extension:* deltoid posterior fibers, latissimus dorsi, pectoralis major, teres major. *Adduction:* latissimus dorsi, pectoralis major, teres major. *Elbow extension:* triceps brachii (SH, LatH), anconeus

Antagonists: *Shoulder extension:* anterior deltoid, coracobrachialis, biceps brachii, pectoralis major. *Shoulder adduction:* supraspinatus, middle deltoid. *Elbow extension:* brachialis, biceps brachii, brachioradialis

Poses: *Contracts:* urdhva dhanurasana. *Lengthens:* purvottanasana

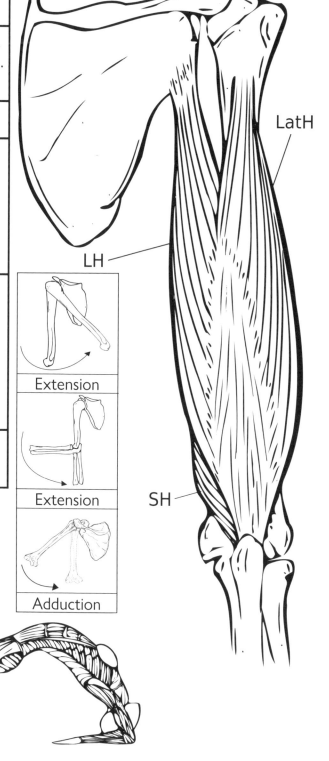

LatH

LH

SH

Extension

Extension

Adduction

FOREARM MUSCLES

The forearm muscles work together to bring the arm into pronation and supination as well as flexion and extension of the wrist. Weak forearm muscles inhibit the ability to support weight from the upper body in poses and movements that bring the weight of the body to the hands. In order to bring strength to the wrists, doing movements and yoga poses that require pronation, supination, wrist flexion, and wrist extension will bring strength to the muscles. Adho mukha svanasana (downward facing dog), bitilasana (cow pose), and marjaryasana (cat pose) are poses that work slowly to strengthen muscles of the wrist. Since the wrist joint is a fragile joint, it is important to become aware of the sensations of the wrists during yoga. If the wrists feel painful, back off from a pose or use yoga props to take some weight off the wrists.

FOREARM MUSCLES

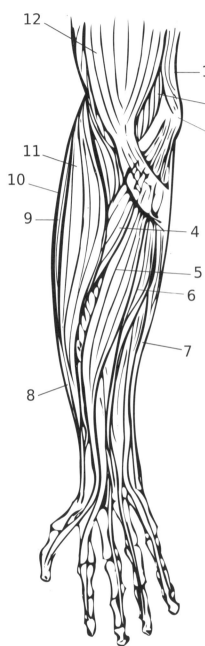

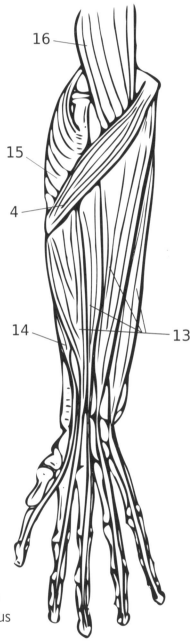

1. Triceps brachii
2. Brachialis
3. Medial epicondyle
4. Pronator teres
5. Flexor carpi radialis
6. Palmaris longus
7. Flexor carpi ulnaris
8. Adductor pollicis longus
9. Extensor carpi radialis brevis
10. Extensor carpi radialis longus
11. Brachioradialis
12. Biceps brachii
13. Flexor digitorium superficialis
14. Flexor pollicis longus
15. Supinator
16. Brachialis

Superficial muscles
reversed

ELBOW FLEXION AND ELBOW EXTENSION

Elbow flexion and extension occurs when muscles contract and relax to bring the forearm towards or away from the upper arm bone. Strong elbow flexors and extensors assist with elbow joint stabilization and help reduce the chance of injury at the elbow joint. It is also important to create strength and balance in the elbow flexors and extensors because, along with the muscles of the shoulders and core, the elbow joint muscles help to load weight from the body when in poses like chaturanga dandasana (four-limbed staff pose) and work to decrease the amount of weight put into the wrist joints.

To activate the elbow flexors
Stand in mountain pose with the palms facing forwards. Engage the core and neutralize the pelvis. Stabilize the scapulothoracic joint. Begin to bend the arm at the elbow while pressing the upper arm bone strongly into the ribcage (adduction). Move slowly until the wrists reach the shoulders.

To activate the elbow extensors
In mountain pose with the arms in a fully flexed position, begin to straighten the arms at the elbow joint while pressing the upper arm bone strongly into the ribcage. Move slowly until the arms are fully straight.

Couple these movements and repeat 5–10 times.

What did you notice? Where did you feel tension? Were you able to create stability and resistance while pressing the arms into the ribcage?

ELBOW FLEXION AND ELBOW EXTENSION

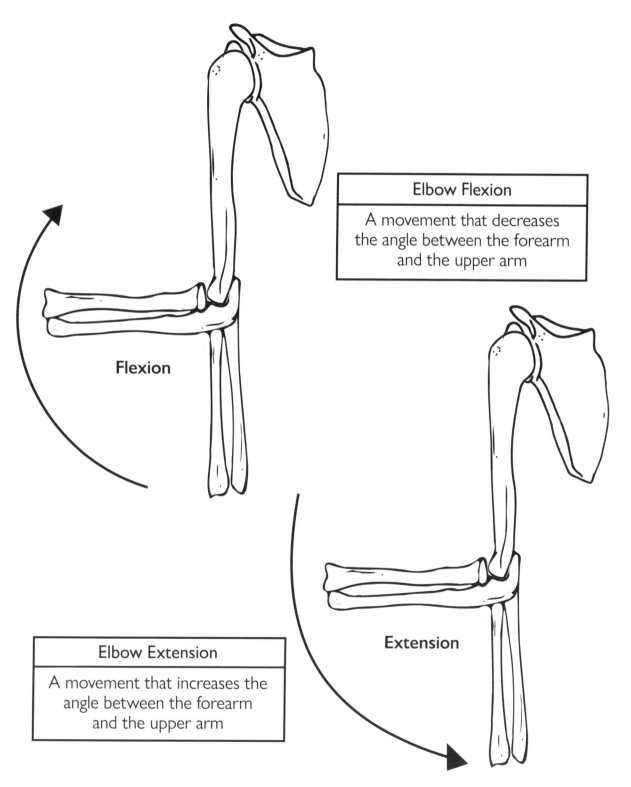

Flexion

Elbow Flexion

A movement that decreases the angle between the forearm and the upper arm

Extension

Elbow Extension

A movement that increases the angle between the forearm and the upper arm

DIAPHRAGM

The diaphragm is a dome-shaped sheet of muscle that separates the thoracic cavity from the abdominal cavity. It gets its unique dome shape from the way it attaches to the spine, ribs, and sternum. The vena cava, aorta, and esophagus run through the diaphragm through separate hiatuses (openings) in the muscles. During inhalation, the diaphragm contracts and pushes the contents of the abdomen down and outwards, making room for the lungs to expand into the chest cavity. During exhalation, as the lungs compress, the diaphragm moves upwards and relaxes back into a resting state.

When functioning properly, the diaphragm is in a harmonious state with the breath. When weak or tight, the harmony can become out of sync and can create a cycle of inefficient breaths. Taking time to connect the mind with the body and breath during pranayama or meditation can help bring awareness to the state of the diaphragm and can help even out any imbalances.

Breath practice

To get in touch with your diaphragm, lie on your back and close your eyes. Turn your focus onto your breath cycle and begin to simply notice it. After a few breaths, start to force a slow and deep exhale out of your lungs. As you do this, feel how your core body contracts to push the air out. At the end of your exhale, hold the tension your core has created for a second. Then, instead of forcing in an inhalation, relax the tension of the core created by the forced exhalation. Practice this for a few minutes and study what effect it has on your breathing cycle.

What did you notice? Did your inhalation naturally follow when you relaxed the tension built from the exhalation? Did your inhalation feel full and easy?

When the tension is released the diaphragm is triggered to contract and push the abdominal contents down and out. Consciously bringing your attention to the moment the core tension releases and the diaphragm contracts helps the diaphragm build strength and rhythm and restores harmony back to the breathing cycle. A harmonious breath is a harmonious mind and body.

DIAPHRAGM

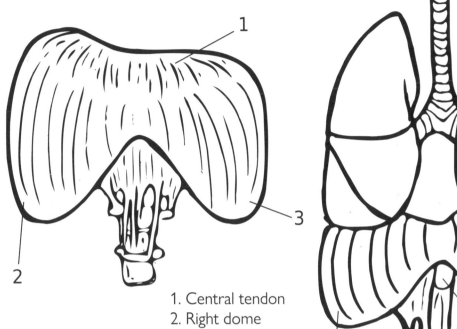

1. Central tendon
2. Right dome
3. Left dome
4. Caval opening
5. Esophageal hiatus
6. Aortic hiatus

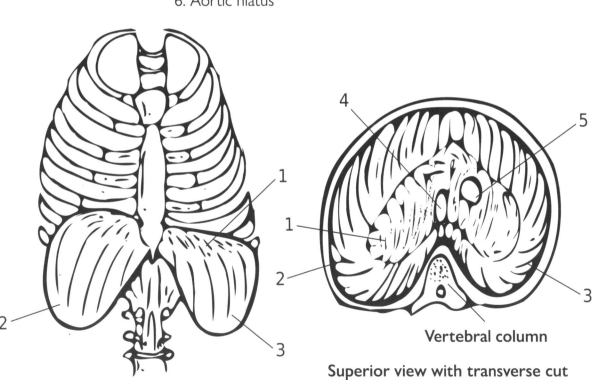

Vertebral column

Superior view with transverse cut

LUNGS

When it comes to yoga asana, the lungs are a big area of focus. Each movement is initiated with a breath, allowing the breath to lead and guide the body into poses. The main reasons for breath are to deliver oxygen to the cells of the body for use in biological functions and to eliminate waste, carbon dioxide, created by the cells during completion of biological functions.

Air enters into the lungs through a pathway. This pathway starts when air is drawn in from the atmosphere and enters into the nasal or oral cavity. The air then travels to the pharnyx and the trachea and branches out into a network of branches called the primary bronchii, located in the right and left lobes of the lungs. From the primary bronchii the air travels to the secondary bronchii, to the tertiary bronchii, and then to the bronchioles—which are the tips of the branched network. Once in the bronchioles, the air is transferred to the alveoli. The alveoli are tiny air sacs and the site where rapid gas exchange occurs. Here, the oxygen diffuses into the blood stream and carbon dioxide diffuses out. Once the oxygen passes into the blood stream it is picked up by hemoglobin. Hemoglobin is a protein in red blood cells that carry oxygen throughout the body. The red blood cells are pumped throughout the body via the heart and deliver the oxygen to cells that are in need. These cells then use the oxygen to create energy in order to perform action. For example, the muscle cells need oxygen and energy in order to produce a contraction. Once the cells complete an action, waste is created in the form of carbon dioxide.

When carbon dioxide is created, it is transferred to the hemoglobin on the red blood cell and is carried through the blood stream to the alveoli of the lungs. The carbon dioxide is diffused out of the blood and enters the network of branches in the lungs, traveling from the bronchioles, to the tertiary bronchii, to the secondary bronchii, and then to the primary bronchii. From there, the carbon dioxide travels through the trachea, the pharnyx, and out through the nasal or oral cavity to diffuse with the atmosphere. This process occurs with every breath taken and is the most important process of human life, for, without it, life would not occur.

LUNGS

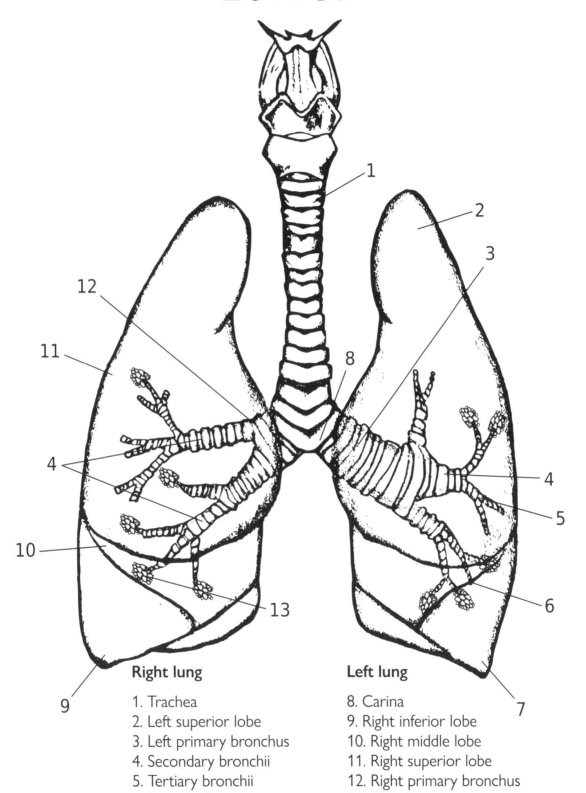

Right lung

1. Trachea
2. Left superior lobe
3. Left primary bronchus
4. Secondary bronchii
5. Tertiary bronchii
6. Bronchioles
7. Left inferior lobe

Left lung

8. Carina
9. Right inferior lobe
10. Right middle lobe
11. Right superior lobe
12. Right primary bronchus
13. Alveoli

PART II
ASANA ANATOMY

APANASANA

Apanasana translates to "wind relieving pose." Apana is the descending energy that flows through the spine, prompting the lungs to exhale waste from the body. Apanasana is originally performed with both knees hugged into the chest. This variation brings length to the extended leg's hip flexors. Inhale to push the bent knee away from the body and exhale to squeeze the leg in towards the chest. Squeezing the leg into the body compresses and awakens the contents of the core body by correlating the breath with the mind and body. As these muscles awaken, they work to provide more support for the lower back and diaphragm. As the knee hugs into the chest, the glutes and quadriceps relax and lengthen. The extended leg presses into the floor, which triggers the glutes to contract and the hip flexors to naturally relax.

Extended leg:

1. The quadriceps contract to extend the leg at the knee joint

2. The iliopsoas lengthens

3. The glutes contract to press the leg into the floor

4. The gastrocnemius contracts to bring the ankle into plantarflexion

Flexed leg:

1a. The iliopsoas and hip flexors contract to flex the leg at the hip joint

2a. The hamstrings contract to flex the leg at the knee joint

3a. The glutes lengthen as the hips flex

4a. The gastrocnemius contracts to bring the ankle joint into plantarflexion

APANASANA

ah-pahn-AHS-uh-nuh
Wind Relieving Pose (Variation)

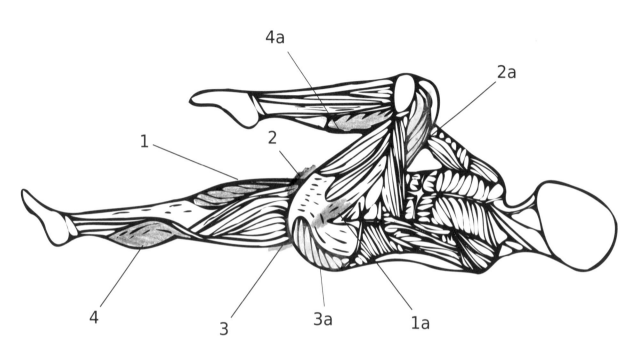

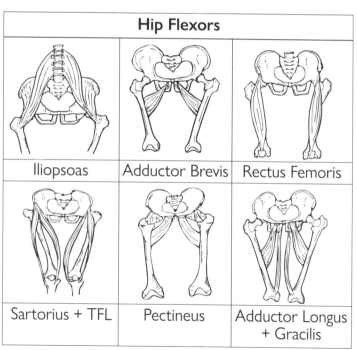

Hip Flexors		
Iliopsoas	Adductor Brevis	Rectus Femoris
Sartorius + TFL	Pectineus	Adductor Longus + Gracilis

SETU BANDHASANA

Setu bandhasana is a gentle inversion that allows the heart to rise higher than the head without putting too much strain onto the body. This pose is known to alleviate stress by calming the brain and central nervous system. As the hips lift in this pose, the glutes contract to support the weight of the pelvis. The shoulder blades retract and the arms extend into the floor. With an easy breath, this pose can bring a sense of relaxation.

Legs:

1. The glutes contract to extend the hips and support the weight of the pelvis

2. The hamstrings contract to flex the knees

3. The quadriceps lengthen

4. The iliopsoas and hip flexors lengthen

5. The adductors engage to stabilize the legs and protect the knees

Trunk:

1b. The rectus abdominis lengthens

2b. The latissimus dorsi contracts to assist with extension of the arms

Arms:

1a. The posterior deltoids contract to extend the arms into the floor

2a. The triceps brachii contracts to extend the elbow joint

3a. The pronators of the forearm contract to press the palms into the floor

4a. The shoulder muscles contract to stabilize the spine on the ribcage

SETU BANDHASANA

SET-too bahn-DAHS-anna

Bridge Pose

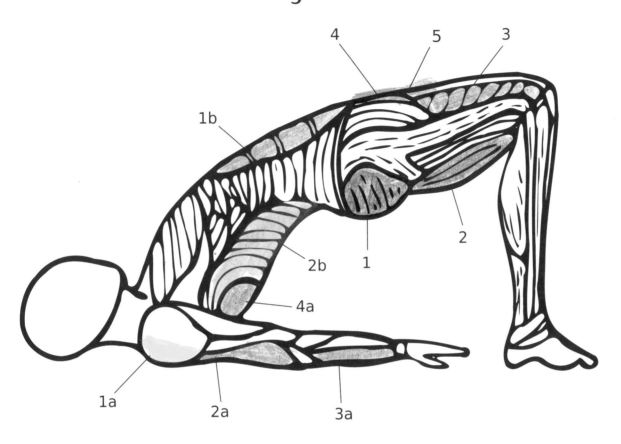

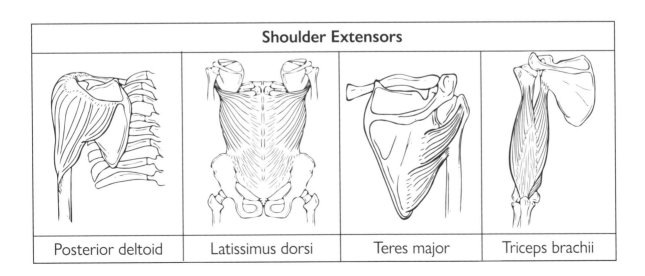

Shoulder Extensors			
Posterior deltoid	Latissimus dorsi	Teres major	Triceps brachii

USTRASANA

With the help of gravitational forces, camel pose opens up the front body while the back body contracts to support and extend the spine into a deep back bend. The posterior deltoid, latissimus dorsi, teres major, infraspinatus, and triceps brachii extend the arms back to grab the heels. The trapezius and rhomboids contract to retract and depress the shoulder blades. This opens up the back of the neck for extension. The erector spinae contract and bring the spine into extension, while the rectus abdominis lengthens and slightly contracts to protect the lumbar spine from hyperextension. The glutes and adductors contract to push the hips forwards while bringing support and stability to the upper body. The lower legs press into the floor to create a strong foundation.

Legs:

1. The glutes contract to extend hips forwards

2. The iliopsoas lengthens as the hips push forwards

3. The hamstrings contract to flex the leg at the knee joint as the shins press into the floor

4. The quadriceps lengthen as the hips push forwards and the knees bend

5. The gastrocnemius contracts as the plantarflexed ankles press into the floor

6. The adductors of the hip contract to bring the legs in towards the midline

Trunk:

1b. The erector spine brings the spine into extension

2b. The quadratus lumborum extends the lumbar spine

3b. The abdominals lengthen as the spine extends and has a slight contraction to protect the spine

Arms:

1a. The posterior deltoids contract to extend the arms at the shoulder joint

2a. The anterior deltoids lengthen as the shoulders extend

3a. The triceps brachii contracts to extend the arms at the elbow joints

4a. The biceps brachii and coracobrachialis lengthen as the elbow extends

5a. The trapezius depresses and retracts the shoulder blades

6a. The rhomboids depress and retract the shoulder blades

7a. The infraspinatus externally rotates the arms at the shoulder joint

8a. The pectoralis muscles lengthen

USTRASANA

oosh-TRAHS-anna

Camel Pose

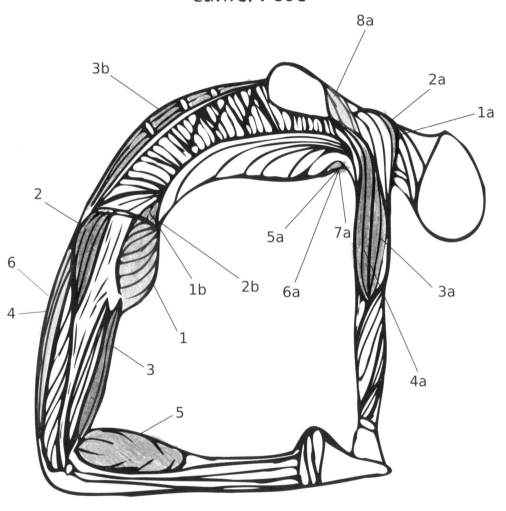

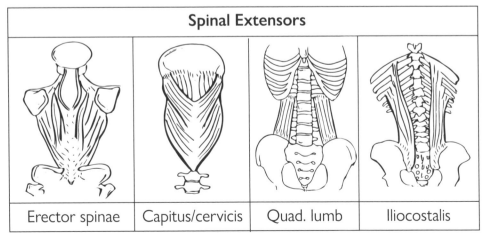

Spinal Extensors			
Erector spinae	Capitus/cervicis	Quad. lumb	Iliocostalis

MARJARYASANA

Marjaryasana (cat pose) is commonly combined with bitilasana (cow pose) which brings the spine into a gentle flexion and extension. Starting with the ankles, the gastrocnemius contracts to press the lower legs and ankle joints into the floor to create a strong connection with the floor. The hamstrings contract to flex the knees while the hip flexors contract to bring flexion to the hips. The rectus abdominis and transversus abdominis activate and bring the spine into flexion. The transverse fibers of the trapezius and rhomboids lengthen as the shoulder blades protract away from each other. The anterior neck muscles contract to bring the cervical spine into flexion.

Legs:

1. The glutes contract to push the hips forwards

2. The iliopsoas contracts to flex the legs at the hip joint

3. The adductors engage to stabilize the hips

4. The hamstrings contract to flex the legs at the knee joint

5. The gastrocnemius contracts to plantarflex the ankle joint as the foot pushes into the floor

Trunk:

1b. The rectus abdominis contracts to bring the spine into flexion

2b. The latissimus dorsi lengthens as the shoulders flex

Arms:

1a. The anterior deltoids contract to flex the arm at the shoulder joint

2a. The triceps brachii contracts to bring the arm into extension at the elbow joint

3a. The flexors of the forearm contract to flex the wrist joint and press the palms into the floor

MARJARYASANA

mhar-jhar-YHAS-anna

Cat Pose

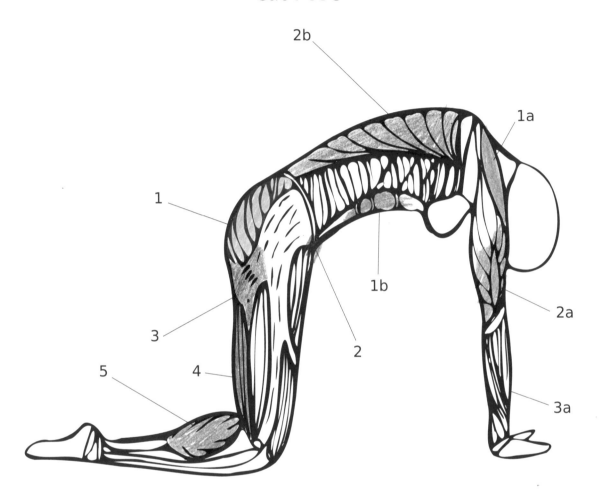

2b

1a

1

1b

3

2

5

4

2a

3a

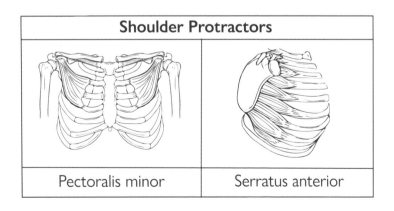

Shoulder Protractors	
Pectoralis minor	Serratus anterior

UTKATASANA

Utkatasana works with gravity to bring strength to the spine and shoulders. The middle deltoids contract to bring the arms into abduction at the shoulder joint. The shoulder blades depress and retract and anchor to the ribcage, providing stability for the arms. The rectus abdominis contracts to stabilize the spine, and the hip flexors deeply contract to flex the hips. While in utkatasana, push your hips back, shift your weight into your heels and try to spread the ground outwards with your feet. These actions are meant to engage your glutes (as the feet try to spread the ground outwards it triggers the gluteus medius to contract). When the glutes contract they support the weight of the pelvis and reduce stress put onto the lower back, knees, and ankles. This variation brings the spine into rotation, allowing for the obliques to strengthen and the opposing obliques to lengthen.

Legs:

1. The iliopsoas and hip flexors deeply contract to flex the legs at the hip joint

2. The quadriceps lengthen to assist the hamstrings in an antagonistic contraction

3. The gastrocnemius contracts to press the feet into the floor

4. The hamstrings contract to flex the knees and support the weight of the thighs

5. The glutes contract to support the weight of the pelvis

Trunk:

1b. The rectus abdominis contracts to stabilize spine

2b. The obliques contract to bring spine into rotation. Opposing side obliques lengthen

Arms:

1a. The middle deltoids contract to bring the arm into abduction

2a. The biceps brachii lengthens as the triceps contract

3a. The trapezius contracts to depress the shoulder blades for shoulder joint stability

4a. The rhomboids draw the shoulder blades together

UTKATASANA

OOT-kah-TAHS-anna

Chair Pose (Variation)

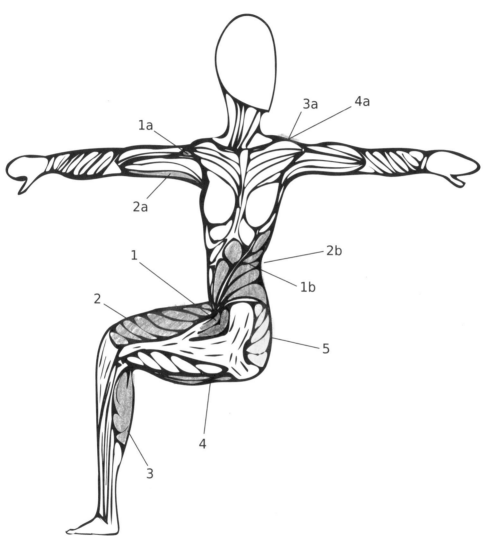

1a

3a   4a

2a

1

1b

2b

2

5

4

3

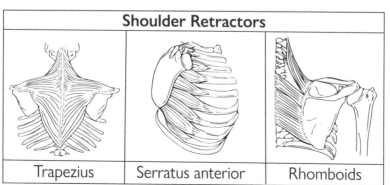

Shoulder Retractors

| Trapezius | Serratus anterior | Rhomboids |

BALASANA

The figure shown in the drawing is entering child's pose in order to provide a better view of the muscles. This resting pose works with gravity to help relax the body into the floor. The quadriceps lengthen to help the hamstrings deeply flex the knees. The hip flexors contract to deeply flex the hips, while the glutes and hip extensors lengthen to assist the hip flexors. The spine lengthens and the anterior deltoids flex the arms forwards. Due to the deep flexing of the hips and the knees, tight hip extensors and knee extensors can inhibit the deep flexion this pose requires. If the hip extensors are tight and this pose brings discomfort, using props under the knees or hips can help increase comfort and reduce pain.

Legs:

1. The iliopsoas contracts deeply to flex the leg at the hip joint

2. The gluteus maximus lengthens

3. The hamstrings contract

4. The quadriceps lengthen

5. The adductors contract to bring the thighs in towards the midline

Trunk:

1b. The abdominals slightly contract to support anterior spine

Arms:

1a. The anterior deltoids contract to bring the shoulder joint into flexion

2a. The triceps contract to extend the arms at the elbow joint

3a. The trapezius contracts to stabilize the shoulder blades

4a. The forearm muscles engage as palms press into the floor

BALASANA

bah-LAHS-anna

Child's Pose

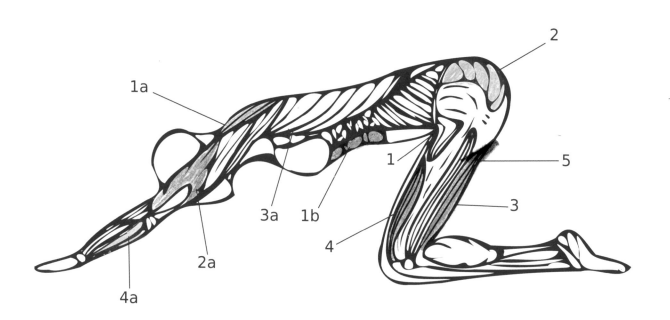

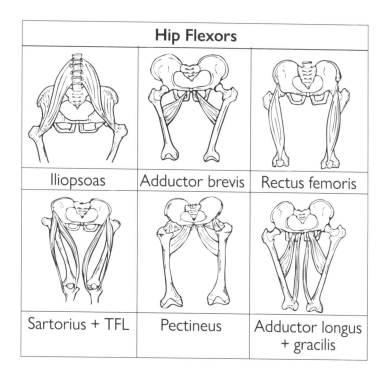

Hip Flexors		
Iliopsoas	Adductor brevis	Rectus femoris
Sartorius + TFL	Pectineus	Adductor longus + gracilis

NATARAJASANA

Natarajasana brings strength and balance to the body and mind. As the standing leg balances and presses into the floor, the gluteus medius is activated to bring strength and stability to the hip joint. The rectus abdominis lengthens and tenses to protect the spine from hyperextending. The posterior deltoid and shoulder extensors contract to send the arm back to reach the foot. This pose brings balance to the mind by requiring a large amount of focus to bring the body into balance.

Legs:

1. The gluteus maximus contracts to extend and lift the leg

2. The iliopsoas and hip flexors lengthen as the leg extends back

3. The adductors and glutes engage to help stabilize the standing leg

4. The lifted leg quadriceps lengthen as the knee flexes

5. The lifted leg hamstrings contract to extend the hips and flex the knee

6. The gastrocnemius contracts and plantarflexes the ankle joint

Trunk:

1b. The rectus abdominis lengthens and tenses to protect the spine from hyperextension

2b. The latissimus dorsi assists in extension of the arm

Arms:

1a. The biceps lengthen while the triceps contract to straighten the arm at the elbow joint

2a. The posterior deltoid extends the arm back to grab the lifted leg ankle joint

3a. The anterior deltoid lengthens

4a. The trapezius muscles contract to depress the shoulder blades

NATARAJASANA
nuh-thar-uh-jah-suh-nuh
Lord of the Dance Pose

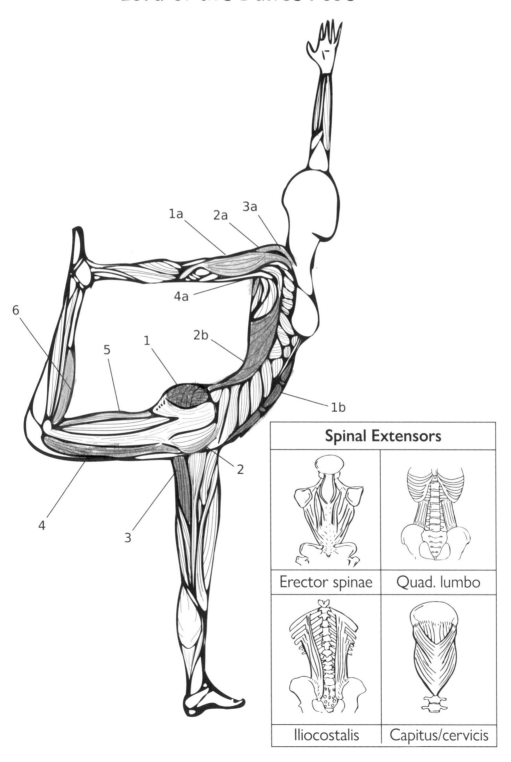

1a 2a 3a

4a

6

1

2b

5

1b

2

4

3

Spinal Extensors

Erector spinae	Quad. lumbo
Iliocostalis	Capitus/cervicis

DHANURASANA

Naturally, as a deep back bending pose, dhanurasana stretches the muscles on the anterior body and contracts and strengthens the muscles on the posterior body. Starting from the shoulder blades, the posterior deltoids contract to extend the arms back to the ankles; this action brings length to the pectoralis muscles. The trapezius contracts to depress the shoulder blades down the back, and the rhomboids contract to bring the shoulder blades in towards the midline, all working together to stabilize the shoulder joint while the hands bind to the ankles. It is important to bring focus to the anterior deltoids and the deep stretch this pose brings to them. If the stretch is uncomfortable, responsible practice encourages releasing your extension. Moving onto the spine, the erector spinae contract to bring the spine into extension, while the rectus abdominis lengthens. During poses that bring a deep extension to the spine, the rectus abdominis also slightly contracts to protect the spine from entering into hyperextension. The hips press into the floor through gluteal contraction, bringing a natural lengthening to the hip flexor muscles. As the hips extend, the quadriceps lengthen while the hamstrings contract to flex the knee joint. The ankles are brought into plantarflexion through contraction of the gastrocnemius. This creates a strong ankle joint for the hands to grab. The inhalation during this pose can be brought into the chest cavity to encourage expansion.

Legs:

1. The hamstrings contract to bring the legs into flexion at the knee joint

2. The glutes contract while the hips press into the floor

3. The quadriceps lengthen

4. The iliopsoas lengthens as the hips extend

5. The gastrocnemius contracts to bring the foot into plantarflexion at the ankle joint

Trunk:

1b. The rectus abdominis lengthens as the spine extends

Arms:

1a. The posterior deltoids contract to extend the arm towards the feet

2a. The triceps contract to bring extension to the elbow joint

3a. The biceps lengthen

4a. The latissimus dorsi contracts as arms extend towards the feet

5a. The pectoralis muscles lengthen as arms extend

DHANURASANA

DON-your-ahs-UN-ah

Bow Pose

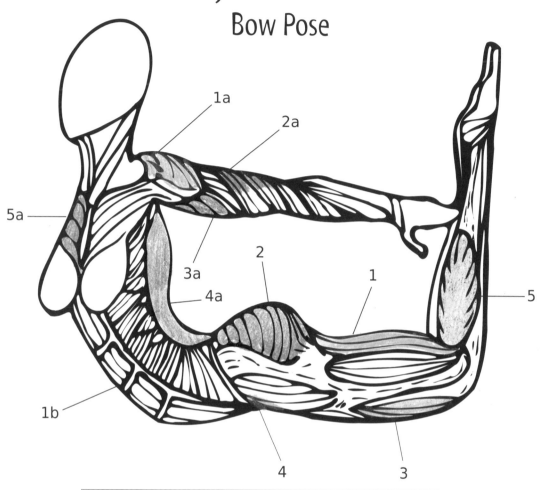

1a
2a
5a
3a
2
1
4a
5
1b
4
3

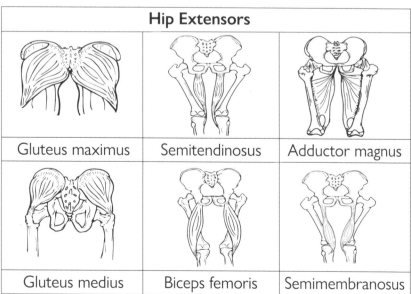

Hip Extensors

Gluteus maximus	Semitendinosus	Adductor magnus
Gluteus medius	Biceps femoris	Semimembranosus

UTTHITA HASTA PADANGUSTHASANA

Utthita hasta padangusthasana requires a stable foundation on one leg (gluteus medius), while needing muscular length in the adductor muscles and muscular strength in the abductor muscles of the lifted leg. Remember to keep the lifted leg bent if pain or discomfort occurs. The standing leg presses into the floor to provide stability for the body. The glutes and iliopsoas contract to stabilize the standing leg, hip joint, and spine. The lifted leg externally rotates and abducts to meet the hand. The gaze fixes and the breath steadies.

Standing leg:

1. The glutes contract to press the foot into the floor

2. The gluteus medius contracts to stabilize the lateral hip

3. The tensor fasciae latae contracts to stabilize the lateral hip

4. The quadriceps contract to extend the leg at the knee joint

5. The tibialis anterior contracts to press the heel of the foot into the floor

6. The gastrocnemius contracts to press the ball of the foot into the floor

Abducted leg:

1a. The abductors of the hip work to bring the leg away from the midline of the body

2a. The adductors of the hip lengthen and assist hip abductors (antagonists)

3a. The iliopsoas and flexors of the hip contract to bring the leg into flexion

4a. The external rotators of the hip externally rotate the leg

5a. The quadriceps contract to extend the leg at the knee joint

6a. The hamstrings lengthen and assist the quadriceps (antagonists)

7a. The tibialis anterior contracts while the foot is in dorsiflexion

Arms:

1b. The middle deltoid contracts to abduct the arm

2b. The external rotators of the shoulder contract

3b. The triceps brachii contracts to extend the arm at the elbow

Trunk:

1c. The abdominals contract to stabilize the anterior spine

2c. The erector spinae contract to stabilize and lengthen the posterior spine

UTTHITA HASTA PADANGUSTHASANA

oo-TEE-tah HA-sta pad-an-goosh-TAHS-anna

Extended Hand–Toe Pose

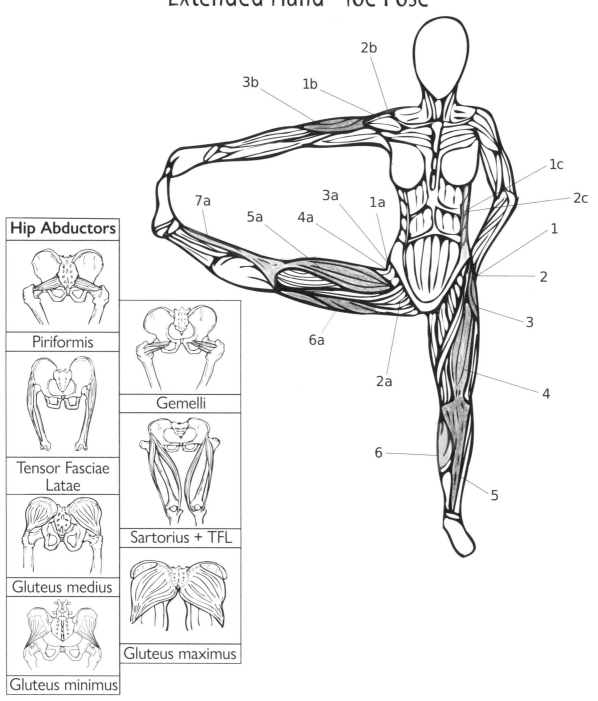

Hip Abductors

Piriformis

Tensor Fasciae Latae

Gluteus medius

Gluteus minimus

Gemelli

Sartorius + TFL

Gluteus maximus

PURVOTTANASANA

A deep extension of the spine strengthens the posterior muscles of the body while lengthening the anterior muscles. The glutes and hip extensors contract to push the hips up and support the weight of the pelvis. The erector spinae contract to bring the back into extension. The anterior deltoids create a strong contraction to flex the arms above the head, while creating a deep stretch in the posterior deltoids. The trapezius and rhomboids depress and retract the shoulder blades and bring support to the shoulder joint. The rectus abdominis lengthens and tenses to protect the lumbar spine. The quadriceps contract to straighten the legs, and the gastrocnemius and soleus calf muscles contract to press the feet into the floor.

Legs:

1. The glutes contract to bring extension to the leg at the hip joint

2. The iliopsoas lengthens and assists the glutes in extension (antagonist)

3. The quadriceps contract to extend the leg at the knee joint

4. The hamstrings slightly contract while the glutes extend to bring the legs into extension at the hip joint

5. The gastrocnemius and soleus contract while the foot pushes into the floor

Trunk:

1b. The rectus abdominis lengthens as the spine is extended

2b. The erector spinae contract and bring the lumbar spine into extension

Arms:

1a. The latissimus dorsi contracts while the arms flex

2a. The posterior deltoids lengthen

3a. The trapezius contracts to depress the shoulder blades down the back

4a. The pectoralis muscles engage while arms squeeze in towards the midline

5a. The biceps contract to bring flexion to the elbow joint

PURVOTTANASANA

pur-voh-than-ahs-ana
Upward Plank Pose (Forearm Variation)

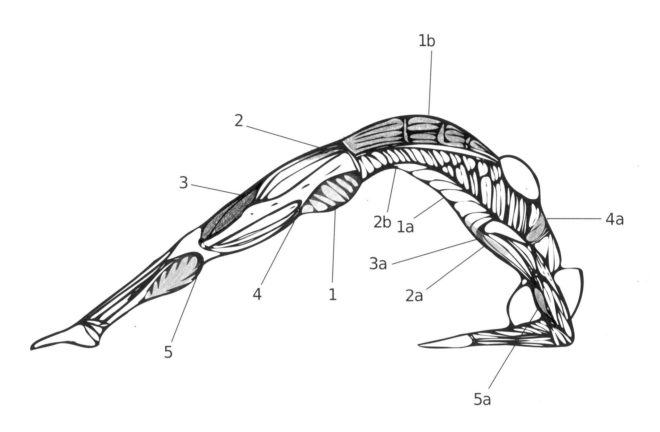

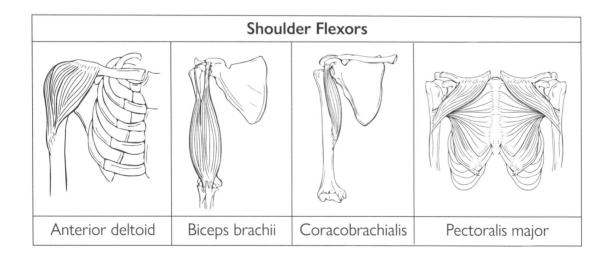

Shoulder Flexors			
Anterior deltoid	Biceps brachii	Coracobrachialis	Pectoralis major

UTKATA KONASANA

Goddess pose brings strength and heat to the hips. The external rotators and abductors of the hips contract and rotate to bring the thighs away from the midline. The iliopsoas and hip flexors squeeze to flex the legs at the hips while also supporting the weight of the trunk. The rectus abdominis and erector spine contract slightly to stabilize the spine. The hamstrings contract and flex the legs at the knee joint while the quadriceps lengthen. The middle fibers of the deltoid contract to abduct the arms away from the midline of the body. While lowering the hips, push the hips out and put your weight into the heels to engage the glutes. Engaging the glutes will bring stability and strength to the hip area.

Legs:

1. The external rotators contract to externally rotate the legs

2. The hamstrings contract to bring the leg into flexion at the knee joint

3. The tibialis anterior contracts to press the feet into the floor

4. The internal rotators lengthen at the hip joint

5. The sartorius externally rotates the thigh

Trunk:

1b. The erector spinae contract to lengthen the spine

2b. The rectus abdominis contracts to protect and stabilize the spine

Arms:

1a. The biceps brachii lengthens as the arm extends

2a. The triceps brachii contracts to extend the arm at the elbow joint

3a. The middle deltoids contract to abduct the arms

4a. The supraspinatus assists to abduct the arms

5a. The rhomboids retract the scapulae in towards the midline of the body

6a. The trapezius contracts to stabilize and depress the shoulder blades

UTKATA KONASANA

oot-kha-tah cone-AHS-anna
Goddess Pose

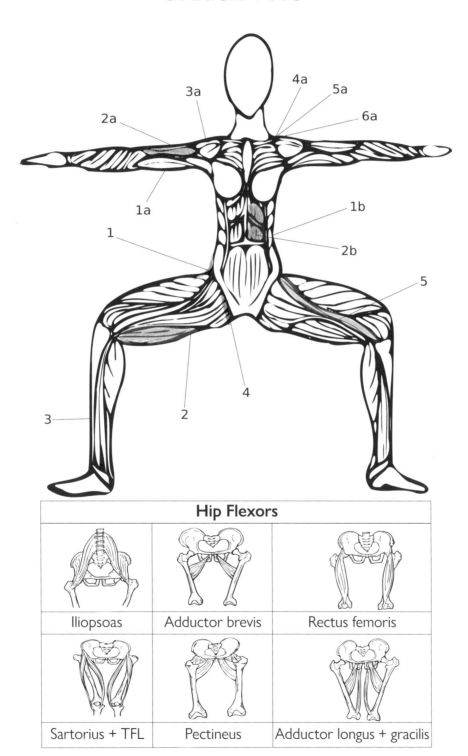

Hip Flexors		
Iliopsoas	Adductor brevis	Rectus femoris
Sartorius + TFL	Pectineus	Adductor longus + gracilis

ARDHA CHANDRASANA

Ardha chandrasana enhances strength, balance, and focus. A strong and stable pelvis will bring feelings of groundedness and stability. The standing leg plants into the floor using the quadriceps and glutes to provide stability to the knee and hip joint. The abductors and external rotators of the hip contract to stack the pelvis and lift the leg. The hip flexors of the standing leg contract to flex the hip forwards. The lifted leg extends back by contracting the glutes and hip extensors. The quadriceps contract to extend and stabilize the lifted leg. As the standing leg hip flexes, the spine is lengthened forwards, using the lateral flexors of the spine to support the weight of the spine and to bring the spine towards the floor. The middle deltoids and shoulder abductors contract to abduct the arms away from the body. The triceps and elbow extensors contract and extend the elbow joint as the hands reach away from the body.

Front leg:

1. The glutes contract to stabilize the pelvis and the head of the femur

2. The abductors of the thigh contract to lift the leg

3. The tibialis anterior contracts to bring the ankle into dorsiflexion

4. The adductors of the thigh stretch

5. The iliopsoas contracts to bring the leg into flexion at the hip joint and to bring balance to the pelvis

Trunk:

1b. The obliques contract to stabilize the spine

2b. The abdominals contract to stabilize the spine

3b. The rhomboids contract and adduct the shoulder blades in towards the spine for shoulder stabilization

Back leg:

1a. The glutes contract to extend and stabilize the leg

2a. The abductors of the thigh contract to lift the leg

3a. The external rotators of the hip contract to externally rotate the leg at the hip joint

4a. The adductors of the thigh stretch

5a. The quadriceps contract to bring the leg into extension at the knee joint

6a. The gastrocnemius lengthens

Arms:

1c. The middle deltoids contract to bring the arm into abduction at the shoulder joint

2c. The trapezius contracts to stabilize the shoulder joint

3c. The triceps contract to extend the arm at the elbow joint

ARDHA CHANDRASANA

ard-HA chan-DRAS-anna

Half Moon Pose

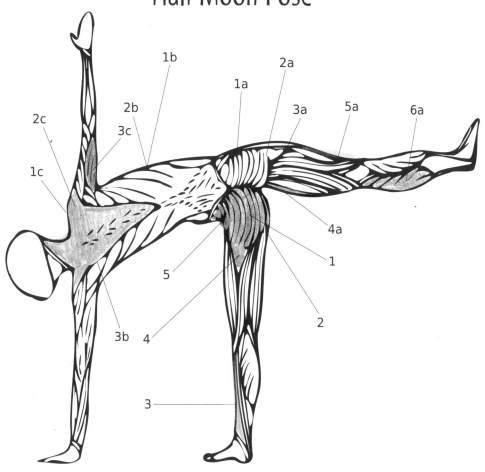

Hip Abductors			
	Gluteus minimus	Gluteus maximus	Gemelli
Sartorius + gracilis	TFL	Piriformis	Gluteus medius

HANUMASANA

Hanumasana is an intense stretch of the hip extensors and the hip flexors. The hip flexors of the front leg strongly contract to bring the leg forwards, giving rise to the intense stretch of the front leg hip extensors. The hip extensors of the back leg strongly contract to extend the leg back, giving rise to an intense stretch of the back leg hip flexors. These actions performed together begin to draw the legs away from each other to lower the pelvis towards the floor. As the pelvis lowers, the hamstrings lengthen while the quadriceps work to straighten the legs into extension. Strong adductors bring the legs in towards the midline and work to stabilize the pelvis. The rectus abdominis and erector spinae contract to stabilize and extend the spine. To avoid injury, it is important to prepare the appropriate muscle groups before trying to enter this pose.

Front leg:

1. The quadriceps contract to extend the leg at the knee joint

2. The hamstrings lengthen to assist the quadriceps in extension

3. The iliopsoas and the hip flexors contract to bring flexion to the hip joint

4. The gluteus maximus lengthens

5. The tensor fasciae latae and the gluteus medius stabilize the lateral hip through internal rotation

Back leg:

1a. The gluteus maximus and hip extensors contract to extend the leg at the hip joint

2a. The tensor fasciae latae and the gluteus medius stabilize the lateral hip through internal rotation

3a. The iliopsoas and the hip flexors lengthen to assist the glutes in extension (antagonists)

4a. The quadriceps contract to extend the leg at the knee joint

5a. The gastrocnemius contracts and brings the ankle joint into plantarflexion and presses the foot into the floor

Arms:

1b. The trapezius contracts to depress the shoulder blades down the back

2b. The anterior deltoids contract to bring flexion to the arms at the shoulder joints

Trunk:

1c. The erector spinae contract to extend the spine

2c. The rectus abdominis contracts to stabilize and protect the spine

HANUMASANA

ha-new-mahn-AHS-anna

Monkey Pose

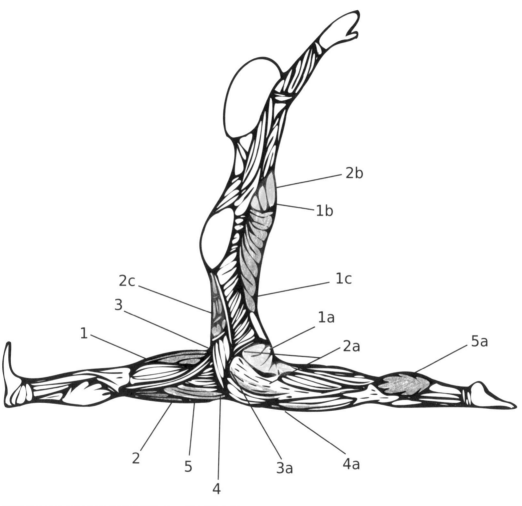

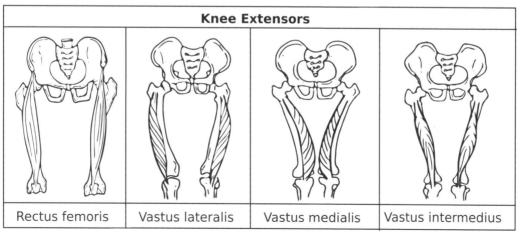

Knee Extensors			
Rectus femoris	Vastus lateralis	Vastus medialis	Vastus intermedius

SALAMBA SIRSASANA

To prevent injury in this pose, developing strength in the shoulder joints is imperative to protect the neck and spine. Strong shoulders create a solid foundation to support the weight of the body. Once the body is strong enough to support itself upside down, maintaining balance is the key focus. While many muscles come into factor to provide balance to the body upside down, the pelvic floor and transversus abdominis plays the biggest role. Bringing focus to the contraction of these muscles brings balance and root strength to the muscles of the core body. As the pelvic floor contracts, the adductors of the hips bring the legs in towards the midline, while the legs reach away from the head. During this pose, the extensors and flexors of the hips and spine activate support and maintain neutral balance of the spine and pelvis.

Legs:

1. The adductors engage to bring the legs in towards the midline

2. The hip flexors engage to provide stability to the front hip

3. The hip extensors engage to provide support to the back hip

4. The quadriceps engage to extend the leg at the knee joint

Trunk:

1b. The muscles of the pelvic floor contract to bring stability to the pelvis and strength to the abdominals

2b. The rectus abdominis contracts to stabilize the front spine

3b. The erector spinae contract to stabilize the back spine

Arms:

1a. The biceps contract to flex the arm at the elbow joint

2a. The anterior deltoids contract to flex the arms at the shoulder joints

3a. The upward rotators of the shoulder blades contract to stabilize the shoulder joint during flexion

SALAMBA SIRSASANA

sah-lham-bah sir-ah-suh-nuh

Supported Headstand

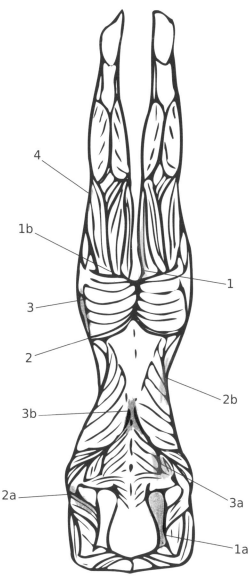

4
1b
3
2
1
2b
3b
2a
3a
1a

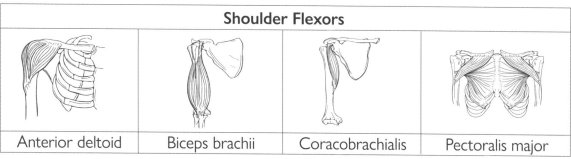

Shoulder Flexors			
Anterior deltoid	Biceps brachii	Coracobrachialis	Pectoralis major

EKA PADA ADHO MUKHA SVANASANA

This downward facing dog variation provides similar benefits to the body as downward dog with the addition of building strength in the extensors of the lifted leg. The external rotators of the shoulder contract to externally rotate the head of the humerus away from the midline of the body. The trapezius contracts to depress and stabilize the shoulder blades, making room behind the neck. The rectus abdominis and pelvic floor muscles contract to protect the spine. The hip flexors of the standing leg squeeze to flex the hips, and the internal rotators of the hips contract to turn the legs inward towards the midline of the body. The quadriceps contract and straighten the leg at the knee joint, and the tibialis anterior contracts to press the heels towards the floor. The lifted leg glutes contract to bring the leg into extension at the hip, and the quadriceps tense to extend the lifted leg.

Legs:

1. The quadriceps contract to straighten the leg at the knee joint

2. The hamstrings lengthen as the quadriceps contract

3. The iliopsoas contracts to flex the legs at the hip joint

4. The pectineus contracts to assist in flexion of the hip joint

5. The sartorius contracts to flex the leg at the hip

6. The tensor fasciae latae and the gluteus medius stabilize the hip joint and internally rotate the legs

7. The glutes contract to extend and lift the leg

Trunk:

1b. The erector spinae contract and extend the lumbar spine

2b. The quadratus lumborum extends the lumbar spine

3b. The abdominals and pelvic floor muscles contract to stabilize and protect the spine

Arms:

1a. The triceps brachii extends the arm at the elbow joint

2a. The hamstrings lengthen as the quadriceps contract

3a. The infraspinatus externally rotates the arms at the shoulder joints

4a. The teres minor externally rotates the arms at the shoulder joints

5a. The rhomboids depress and retract the shoulder blades

6a. The trapezius depresses and retracts the shoulder blades

EKA PADA ADHO MUKHA SVANASANA

eh-kah pah-dah ah-doh MOO-kuh

shvan-AHS-anna

One-Legged Downward Dog

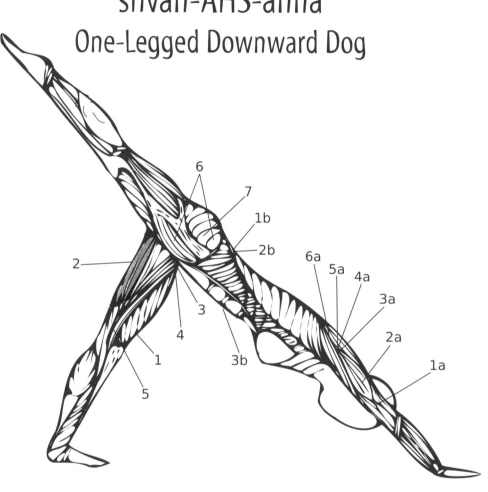

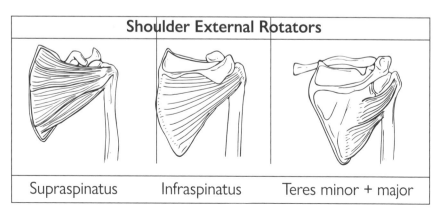

Shoulder External Rotators		
Supraspinatus	Infraspinatus	Teres minor + major

HALASANA

Usually performed after shoulder stand, halasana is a pose that opens up the back of the body. The posterior fibers of the deltoids and triceps contract to extend and press the arms into the floor. The trapezius contracts and depresses the shoulder blades down the back, making length for the back of the neck to extend. The back of the head presses into the floor to protect the cervical spine, and the thoracic and lumbar spine lengthen and flex as the legs are brought over the head. The hip flexors contract and bring the legs over the head while the quadriceps work to extend the legs at the knee.

Legs:

1. The iliopsoas and hip flexors squeeze to stabilize and flex the hips

2. The pectineus contracts to assist with hip flexion

3. The hip adductors contract to adduct the thighs in towards the midline

4. The quadriceps contract to bring the legs into extension at the knee joint

5. The hamstrings lengthen

Trunk:

1b. The quadratus lumborum contracts to stabilize the lumbar spine

2b. The abdominals and pelvic floor muscles contract to balance and stabilize the spine

3b. The erector spinae contract to stabilize and lengthen the spine

Arms:

1a. The posterior fibers of the deltoid contract to bring the shoulder into extension and press the arms into the floor

2a. The adductors of the shoulder contract to bring the arms in towards the midline

3a. The trapezius contracts to depress the shoulder blades

4a. The rhomboids contract to retract the shoulder blades

5a. The triceps brachii contracts to extend the arm at the elbow joint and press the arms into the floor

6a. The forearm flexors engage to press the hands into the floor

HALASANA

hah-LAHS-anna
Plow Pose

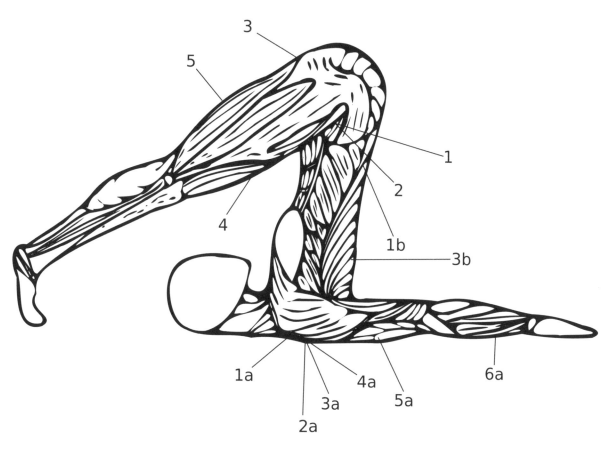

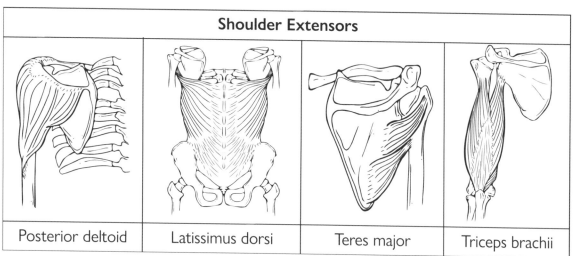

Shoulder Extensors			
Posterior deltoid	Latissimus dorsi	Teres major	Triceps brachii

PARSVOTTANASANA

Parsvottanasana intensely lengthens the hamstrings as the hips flex and the quadriceps contract to straighten the legs at the knee joint. The hip adductors engage to bring the legs in towards the midline, providing stability to the pelvis. The hip flexors contract to bend the trunk forwards. The glutes and hip extensors open and lengthen as the hips flex. The rectus abdominis contracts and flexes the spine forwards towards the feet, bringing a long stretch to the extensors of the spine, the erector spinae. Depending on the arm variation in this pose, the anterior fibers of the deltoids flex the arms at the shoulder joint while the triceps extend the elbow joint, lengthening the forearms towards the floor. The narrow stance of this pose creates a need for focus and balance. If the body feels comfortable and the hip flexors are strong and stable, the flexion of the spine can be deepened for a more intense posterior side stretch. If the body feels unbalanced the stance can widen.

Legs:

1. The iliopsoas contracts to flex the hips

2. The gluteus maximus lengthens as the hips flex

3. The hamstrings lengthen as the hips flex

4. The quadriceps contract and straighten both knees

5. The gastrocnemius lengthens on the back leg

Trunk:

1b. The rectus abdominis flexes the trunk forwards

Arms:

1a. The trapezius depresses the shoulder blades down the back

2a. The rhomboids pull the shoulder blades down the back

3a. The anterior deltoids contract to flex the arms at the shoulder joints

4a. The triceps brachii contracts to extend the arms at the elbow joint

PARSVOTTANASANA

parsh-voh-than-AHS-anna

Intense Side Stretch

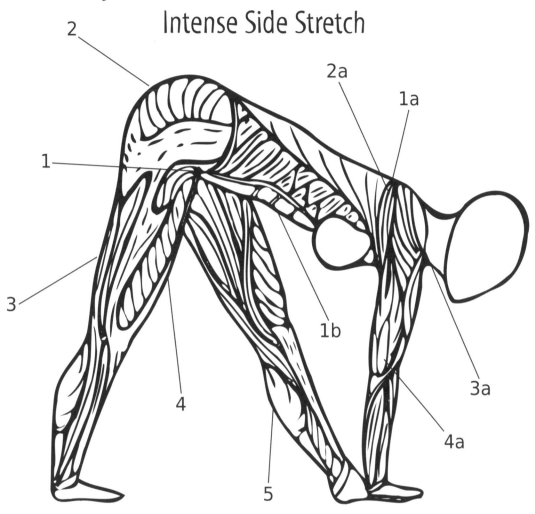

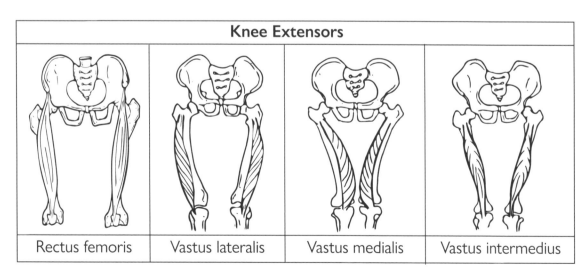

Knee Extensors			
Rectus femoris	Vastus lateralis	Vastus medialis	Vastus intermedius

PARSVA URDHVA HASTASANA

A standing side bend pose allows the spine to flex and lengthen the lateral flexors of the spine. The lateral flexors run along both sides of the spine, working to oppose each other. For example, when the obliques on the right side contract, the obliques on the left side lengthen. These muscles are responsible for stabilizing the spine during spinal flexion as well. In parsva urdhva hastasana, the spine lengthens and laterally bends and brings a refreshed and renewed energy to the spine. The muscles responsible for abducting the shoulder also get a chance to lengthen when the arm is brought over the head.

Legs:

1. The quadriceps contract to extend the leg at the knee joint

2. The glutes contract to stabilize the pelvis and to press the leg into the floor

Trunk:

1b. The internal and external obliques work together with the lateral flexors to contract and bring the spine into lateral flexion

2b. The internal and external obliques and lateral flexors of the spine (opposing side) lengthen to assist in bringing the spine into lateral flexion

3b. The rectus abdominis and transversus abdominis contract to support the anterior spine and firm the organs of the abdominal cavity

Arms:

1a. The trapezius contracts to depress the shoulder blades down the back

2a. The rhomboids contract to retract and stabilize the shoulder blades

3a. The triceps brachii lengthens the arm at the elbow joint

4a. The anterior and middle fibers of the deltoid contract to flex and abduct the arm at the shoulder joint

PARSVA URDHVA HASTASANA

parsva OORD-vah hah-stah-sanna
Upward Salute Pose

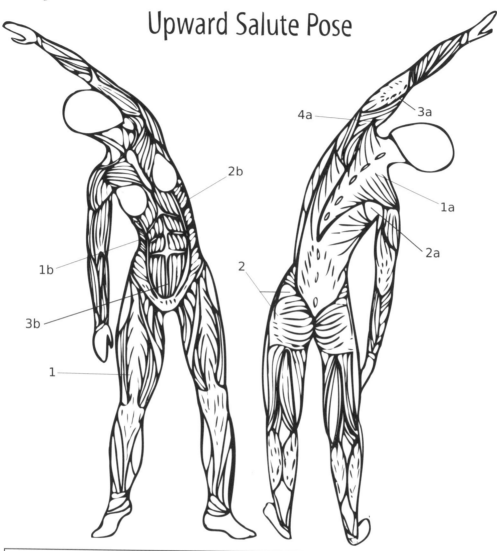

Lateral Flexors			
Internal obliques	External obliques	Quad. lumb	Iliocostalis
Erector spinae	Rectus abdominis	Iliopsoas	Latiss. dorsi

SALAMBA BHUJANGASANA

Sphinx pose brings the spine into a gentle extension, working to strengthen the deep muscles of the spine while opening the muscles of the anterior body. The forearm flexors contract as the palms press into the floor. The posterior deltoids contract to extend the arms at the shoulder joints and pull the forearms back against the floor to further extend the thoracic spine and open the chest. The glutes and adductors of the hips, along with the pelvic floor muscles, contract to press the hips into the floor, rooting the lower body. The quadriceps and gastrocnemius contract to press the legs into the floor.

Legs:

1. The gluteus maximus and hip adductors contract to press the hips into the floor

2. The iliopsoas lengthens across the hip joint

3. The gastrocnemius contracts and plantarflexes the ankles into the floor

Trunk:

1b. The abdominals lengthen and slightly contract to protect the spine as it extends

2b. The erector spinae contract to bring the spine into extension

Arms:

1a. The posterior deltoids contract to pull the ams back as the thoracic spine extends and opens forwards

2a. The biceps brachii contracts to bring the arms into flexion at the elbow joint

3a. The forearm muscles engage as the palms press into the floor

SALAMBA BHUJANGASANA

sah-lum-bah boo-jahn-g-AHS-ana

Sphinx Pose

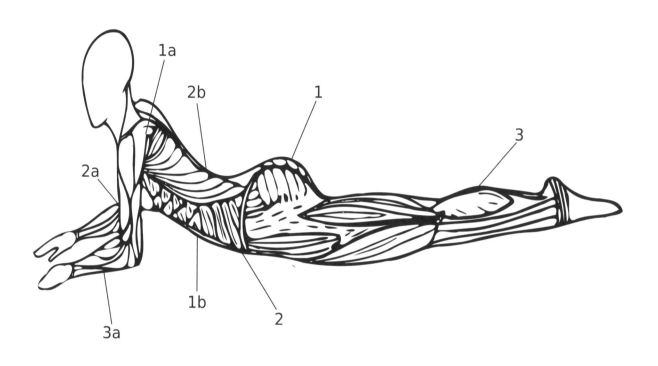

1a
2b
1
2a
3
1b
2
3a

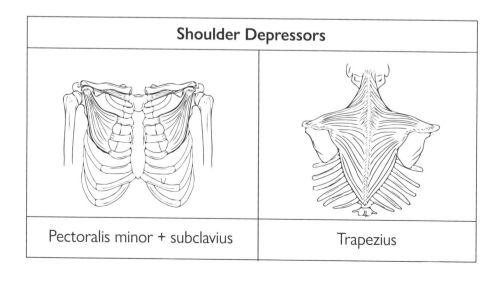

Shoulder Depressors

| Pectoralis minor + subclavius | Trapezius |

UPAVESASANA

Upavesasana requires deep flexion of the hip flexors and length in the hip extensor muscles. The adductors of the hips engage during hip flexion as the knees squeeze in towards the midline to bring balance and stability to the pelvis. Engaging the hip adductors also inhibits the legs from going into abduction too deeply. As the pelvis drops towards the floor, the spine is supported by the rectus abdominis. This pose can be used to awaken the hip flexors and adductors for other poses.

Legs:

1. The iliopsoas and hip flexors deeply contract to bring the hip joint into flexion

2. The hamstrings contract to bring flexion to the knee joint

3. The quadriceps relax to assist the hamstrings in flexion of the knee joint

Trunk:

1b. The abdominals contract to stabilize the spine

2b. The erector spinae contract to stabilize the spine

Arms:

1a. The triceps contract to bring the arms into extension at the elbow joint

2a. The biceps relax to assist the triceps in extension of the elbow joint

3a. The rhomboids stabilize and adduct the shoulder blades

4a. The trapezius contracts to depress and stabilize the shoulder joint

UPAVESASANA

oo-pah-ve-SHAHS-anna
Squat Pose

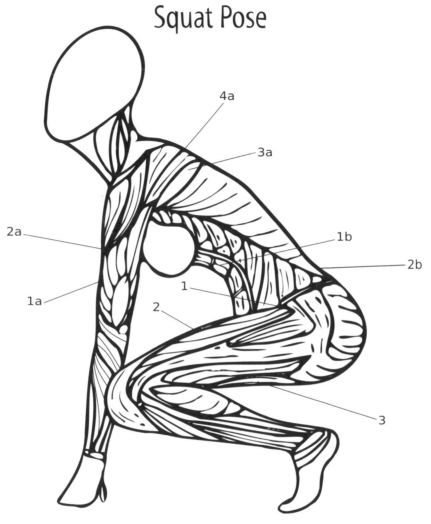

Hip Adductors				
Adductor longus + gracilis	Pectineus	Gluteus maximus	Adductor longus	Adductor brevis

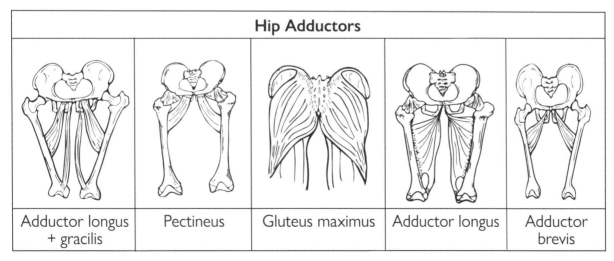

ARDHA UTTANASANA

In the standing half forwards fold, the hip flexors contract to pull the pelvis and spine forwards. The hip extensors assist this movement by lengthening. If the hip extensors are tight, or the hip flexors are weak, the hips may be unable to flex deeply. The quadriceps engage to extend and stabilize the knee joint and the feet press into the floor. This may cause an uncomfortable bend in the spine. To make sure the spine is straight, the knees can flex in this pose.

Legs:

1. The hamstrings lengthen as the quadriceps and hip flexors contract

2. The quadriceps contract to extend the knee joint

3. The iliopsoas and rectus femoris contract and pull the pelvis into flexion

4. The glutes and hip extensors lengthen as the pelvis flexes forwards

Trunk:

1b. The rectus abdominis and pelvic floor muscles contract to stabilize the lower spine and assist in the flexion of the hips

Arms:

1a. The rhomboids and shoulder adductors medially draw in the shoulder blades

2a. The trapezius and shoulder depressors depress the shoulder blades

ARDHA UTTANASANA
ARD-huh ooh-tuhn-AHS-uh-nuh
Standing Half Forward Bend

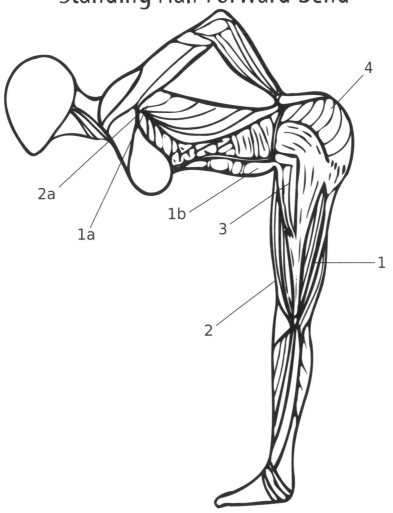

Knee Extensors			
Rectus femoris	Vastus lateralis	Vastus medialis	Vastus intermedius

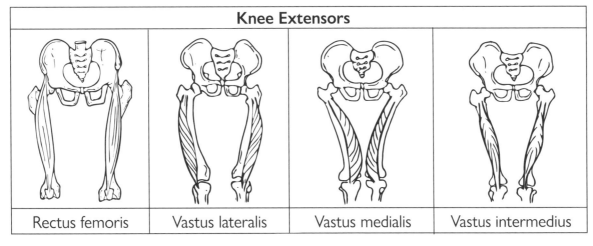

JATHARA PARIVRTTI

Supine belly twists are poses that bring a rotational action to the spine, allowing for the extensors and flexors of the spine to lengthen evenly. The pectoralis muscles and the shoulder adductors lengthen when the arm is outstretched. The hip flexors of the flexed leg contract allowing the hip extensors to lengthen. The hip extensors of the bottom leg contract and stabilize the leg. This supine twist can be practiced after poses that bring the spine into deep flexion or extension, since the action of a spinal twist can gently reset the spinal muscles.

Extended leg:

1. The iliopsoas lengthens

2. The glutes contract to stabilize the pelvis and extend the leg at the hip joint

3. The quadriceps contract to straighten the leg at the knee joint

4. The gastrocnemius contracts during plantarflexion of the ankle joint

5. The tibialis anterior stretches during plantarflexion of the ankle joint

Flexed leg:

1a. The hamstrings contract

2a. The quadriceps lengthen

3a. The glutes and hip extensors lengthen

4a. The adductors of the thigh contract to bring the leg in towards the midline

Arms:

1b. The triceps contract to extend the arm at the shoulder joint

2b. The biceps relax to assist the triceps in extension of the elbow joint

3b. The middle deltoids contract to bring the arm into abduction

4b. The rhomboids contract to bring the shoulder blades medially towards the spine

5b. The trapezius contracts to depress the shoulder blades

Trunk:

1c. The internal and external obliques lengthen

2c. The upper abdominals lengthen

3c. The pectoral muscles lengthen as the arm abducts

JATHARA PARIVRTTI

AT-hara par-ee-VRIT-ti
Belly Twist (Variation)

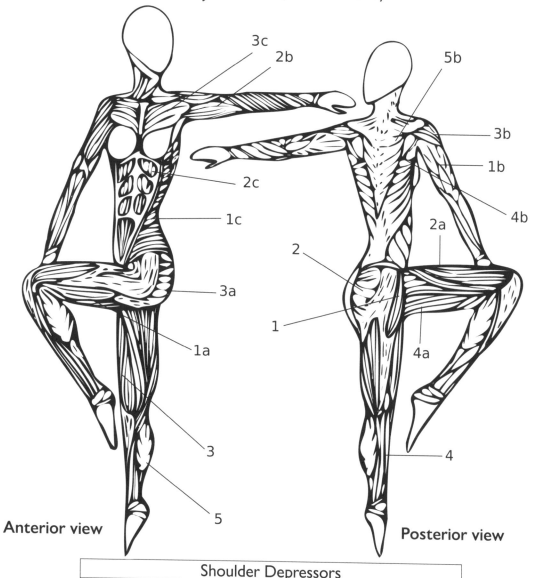

3c
2b
2c
1c
3a
1a
3
5

Anterior view

5b
3b
1b
4b
2a
2
1
4a
4

Posterior view

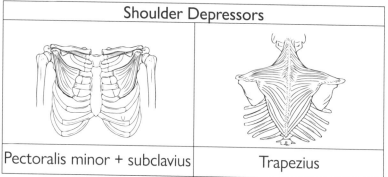

Shoulder Depressors

| Pectoralis minor + subclavius | Trapezius |

TADASANA

In tadasana, the body is in what is considered to be "the anatomical position" in the anatomy world. This position is used to reference body parts in relation to one another. In yoga, tadasana is the starting pose for most standing positions and usually the pose is used to start off yoga classes. It allows the body and mind to take a moment to connect before the practice of asana. During tadasana, the glutes and quadriceps slightly contract as the legs press down into the floor. The inner thighs are drawn towards each other as the adductors engage. The rectus abdominis and erector spinae work together to support the neutral spine, and the anterior muscles of the neck contract to lengthen the posterior side of the neck. The shoulder blades fix to the ribcage, and the external rotators and forearm supinators contract to turn the palms forwards.

Legs:

1. The glutes engage to press the feet into the floor

2. The quadriceps engage to stabilize the knee joint

Trunk:

1b. The rectus abdominis and pelvic floor muscles engage to stabilize the spine

2b. The erector spinae engage to stabilize the spine

3b. The anterior neck muscles engage to draw the chin down slightly

Arms:

1a. The external rotators of the shoulder contract to externally rotate the arm

2a. The forearm muscles contract to supinate the forearm to face the palms forwards

TADASANA

tah-dah-suh-nuh
Mountain Pose

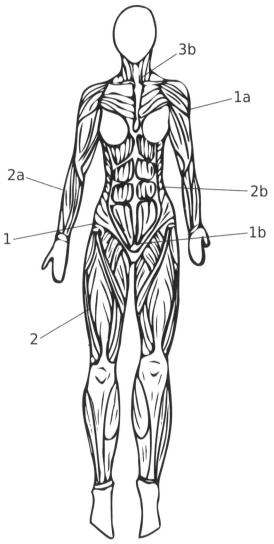

3b

1a

2a

2b

1

1b

2

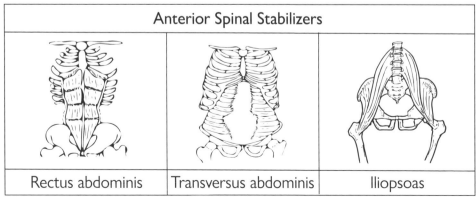

Anterior Spinal Stabilizers		
Rectus abdominis	Transversus abdominis	Iliopsoas

UTTHITA TRIKONASANA

During triangle pose, the front hip flexes forwards and the quadriceps contract to extend the knee. This brings deep lengthening to the hamstrings. The external rotators turn the femur bone away from the midline. The abductors of both hips contract to push the legs away from the midline, creating torque to rotate the spine and open the chest. The rectus abdominis and erector spinae work together to stabilize the spine in a neutral position. The middle deltoids and the abductors of the scapula contract to bring the shoulders away from the midline. The triceps extend the arms at the elbow joint as the hands reach in opposite directions.

Front leg:

1. The iliopsoas contracts and brings the hip joint into flexion

2. The quadriceps contract to extend the leg at the knee joint

3. The glutes and hip extensors lengthen

4. The hamstrings deeply lengthen

5. The gastrocnemius contracts as the foot presses into the floor

Back leg:

1a. The hip extensors slightly engage

2a. The quadriceps contract to extend the leg at the knee joint

3a. The tibialis anterior contracts to bring the foot into dorsiflexion at the ankle joint

4a. The hamstrings lengthen

Arms:

1b. The shoulder abductors contract to push the shoulder blades away from the midline

2b. The middle deltoids contract to abduct the arm at the shoulder joint

3b. The triceps extend the arm at the elbow joint

Trunk:

1c. The obliques contract to rotate the trunk upward towards the ceiling

2c. The erector spinae assist in rotation of the trunk

3c. The abdominals contract to stabilize the spine

UTTHITA TRIKONASANA

oo-TE-tah trik-cone-AHS-anna

Extended Triangle Pose

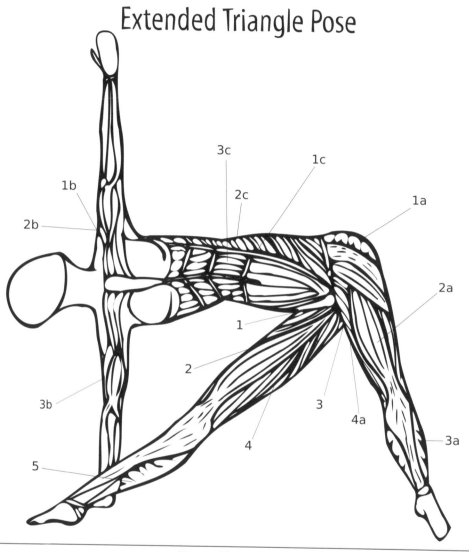

3c
1c
2c
1b
2b
1a
2a
1
2
3
4a
3b
4
3a
5

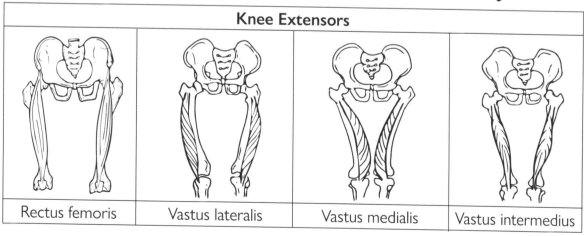

Knee Extensors

| Rectus femoris | Vastus lateralis | Vastus medialis | Vastus intermedius |

VIPARITA KARANI

Viparita karani brings the feet higher than the head, allowing for fluids to drain from the feet and legs, often bringing on a sense of restoration. In this pose, the anterior muscles of the neck contract to flex the cervical spine and, at the same time, the head presses down into the floor and the cervical extensors activate in order to protect the posterior side of the cervical spine. The rhomboids and external rotators of the shoulder work to stabilize the shoulder blades while the spine and pelvis are supported by the hands. The hip flexors contract to lift the legs, and the hip extensors contract to stabilize the lifted legs. The quadriceps contract and extend the knees.

Arms:

1. The biceps brachii contracts to flex the arm at the elbow joint

2. The brachialis assists in flexion of the arm at the elbow joint

3. The posterior deltoids contract to extend the arms at the shoulder joints and press the arms into the floor

4. The rhomboids contract and adduct the shoulder blades inward towards the midline

5. The infraspinatus externally rotates the arm at the shoulder joint

6. The teres minor externally rotates the arm at the shoulder joint

Trunk:

1b. The rectus abdominis contracts to stabilize the spine

2b. The erector spinae contract to extend and stabilize the lumbar spine

3b. The anterior neck muscles contract to bring flexion to the cervical spine

Legs:

1a. The gluteus maximus contracts and stabilizes the posterior pelvis

2a. The iliopsoas contracts and stabilizes the anterior pelvis

3a. The adductors bring the legs in towards the midline

4a. The tensor fasciae latae stabilizes the lateral side of the pelvis

5a. The gluteus medius stabilizes the lateral side of the pelvis

6a. The quadriceps contract and extend the leg at the knee joint

VIPARITA KARANI
vip-par-ee-tah car-AHN-ee
Inverted Pose

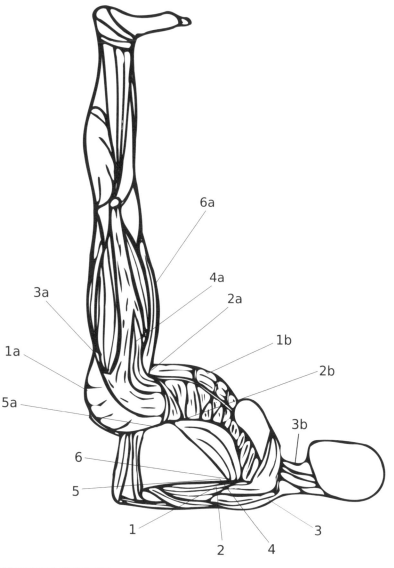

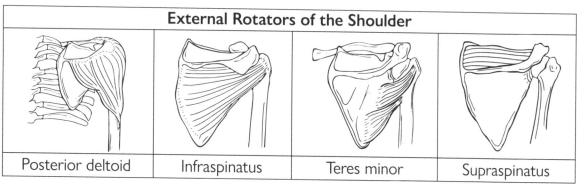

External Rotators of the Shoulder			
Posterior deltoid	Infraspinatus	Teres minor	Supraspinatus

VIRABHADRASANA I

Known as warrior I, virabhadrasana I lengthens the back leg iliopsoas and hip flexors while strengthening the front leg hip flexors and hamstring muscles. The spine lengthens as the arms come into full abduction and flexion. Due to the narrow stance of this pose, when practiced, it strengthens the muscles for balance. If balancing in this pose is too difficult, it is customary to widen the base of support to gain more balance.

Front leg:

1. The quadriceps lengthen

2. The hamstrings contract to bring flexion to the knee

3. The iliopsoas and hip flexors contract to stabilize and flex the hips

4. The pectineus contracts to aid in hip flexion (deep)

5. The tensor fasciae latae and gluteus maximus contract to bring stabilization to the hip in a flexed position

Back leg:

1a. The glute muscles contract to extend the back leg

2a. The iliopsoas and hip flexors relax to aid in hip extension

3a. The quadriceps contract to extend and stabilize the leg at the knee joint

4a. The tibialis anterior contracts to dorsiflex the ankle

5a. The gastrocnemius lengthens during dorsiflexion of the ankle

6a. The hamstrings contract to stabilize the hip in extension

Arms:

1b. The biceps brachii stretches to aid the elbow in extension (antagonist)

2b. The triceps contract to bring the elbow into extension

3b. The anterior deltoids contract to extend the arms at the shoulder joint

4b. The trapezius contracts to depress the shoulder blades

5b. The serratus anterior contracts to upwardly rotate the scapula

Trunk:

1c. The pectoralis major and minor lengthen

2c. The quadratus lumborum and the erector spinae contract to stabilize the posterior spine (deep)

3c. The rectus abdominis and pelvic floor muscles engage to stabilize the anterior spine

VIRABHADRASANA I

veer-ah-bah-DRAHS-anna

Warrior I

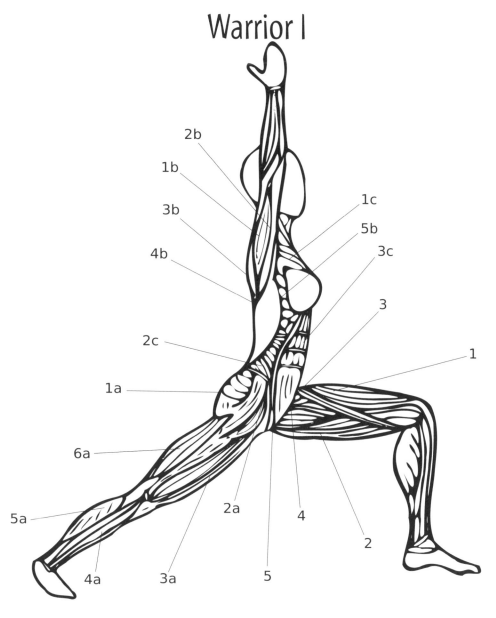

Hip Extensors		
Gluteus maximus	Semitendinosus	Adductor magnus

VIRABHADRASANA II

Starting with the arms, the middle fibers of the deltoid work together with the abductors and upward rotators of the scapula to bring the arms away from the midline. The triceps brachii and elbow extensors engage to bring extension to the forearm, and the pronators of the forearm contract to face the palms downward. Moving down the body, the rectus abdominis and erector spinae contract slightly to support the neutral spine. The abductors of the hips contract and open the hips. The back leg quadriceps and glutes contract to extend the leg. And the external rotators of the hip rotate the back leg open. The hamstrings and hip flexors contract to flex the front leg at the knee and hip.

Front leg:

1. The iliopsoas contracts to flex the leg at the hip joint (deep)

2. The pectineus aids in hip flexion (deep)

3. The sartorius brings stability to the flexed hip

4. The gastrocnemius and soleus contract as the front foot pushes into the floor

5. The hip adductors lengthen during external rotation and abduction of the hip

Arms:

1b. The middle fibers of the deltoids contract to abduct the arm at the shoulder joint

2b. The supraspinatus abducts the arm the first 15 degrees

3b. The rhomboids adduct the shoulder blades medially for joint stabilization

4b. The trapezius slightly adducts and depresses the shoulder blades to stabilize the shoulder joint

5b. The triceps contract to extend the arm at the shoulder joint

Back leg:

1a. The gluteus muscles bring the leg into extension

2a. The adductor magnus stabilizes the leg and aids in extension

3a. The tensor fasciae latae and gluteus medius work together to stabilize the head of the femur during external rotation of the leg

4a. The quadriceps contract to bring the knee joint into extension

5a. The tibialis anterior dorsiflexes the ankle

Trunk:

1c. The rectus abdominis contracts to stabilize the anterior neutral spine

2c. The erector spinae lengthen and stabilize the posterior neutral spine

3c. The quadratus lumborum contracts to stabilize the neutral spine

VIRABHADRASANA II
veer-ah-bah-DRAHS-anna
Warrior II

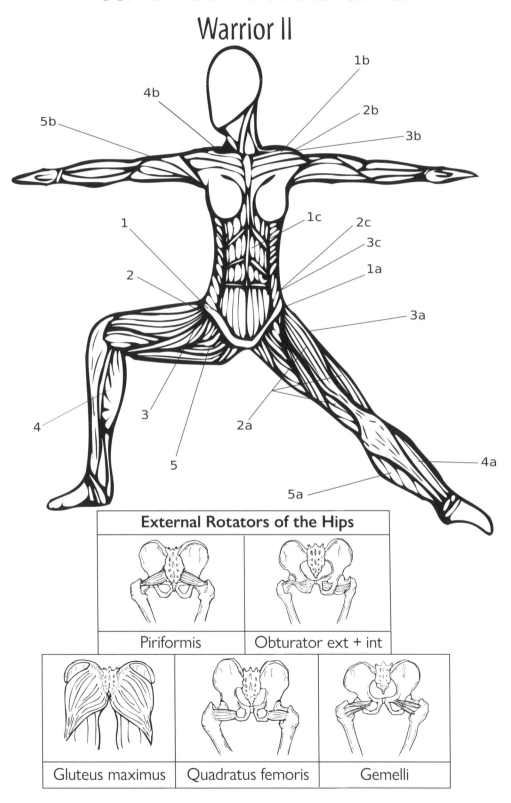

External Rotators of the Hips

Piriformis	Obturator ext + int

Gluteus maximus	Quadratus femoris	Gemelli

URDHVA DHANURASANA

Urdhva dhanurasana is a pose that brings a deep extension to the spine. Starting with the shoulders, anterior deltoids, and shoulder flexors, bring the arm into full flexion and create the base of shoulder support. The rhomboids and shoulder blade adductors bring the shoulder blades medially towards the midline, stabilizing the shoulder joint and supporting the thoracic spine. The serratus anterior slightly contracts to bring further stabilization to the shoulder joint, and the triceps contract to extend the arms at the elbow joint. The pronator muscles of the forearms contract and press the palms into the floor. The erector spinae contract to bring the spine into full extension. While also lengthening, the rectus abdominis slightly contracts to protect the spine from hyperextending. The hip extensors engage to push the pelvis up against gravity, causing the hip flexors to lengthen. The hamstrings contract and bring flexion to the knee joint. Keeping the breath calm and natural will increase comfort during this pose.

Legs:

1. The glutes contract to push the hips against gravity and support the weight of the pelvis

2. The hamstrings work to extend the hips and support the pelvis

3. The tensor fasciae latae contract to stabilize the hip joint

4. The gluteus medius contracts to stabilize the hip joint

5. The tibialis anterior contracts to press the balls of the feet into the floor

6. The gastrocnemius and soleus (deep) lengthen as the balls of the feet press into the floor

Trunk:

1b. The erector spinae contract to bring the spine into extension

2b. The quadratus lumborum and iliopsoas contract to stabilize the lumbar spine while in extension

3b. The rectus abdominis lengthens and slightly contracts to protect the spine

Arms:

1a. The triceps contract to straighten the arm at the elbow joint

2a. The anterior deltoids flex the arms past the head

3a. The pronators of the forearm contract and pronate the forearm

4a. The trapezius contracts to depress the shoulders down the back and stabilize the shoulder joints

5a. The extensors of the forearm extend the wrists

URDHVA DHANURASANA

OORD-vah don-your-AHS-anna

Upward Bow Pose

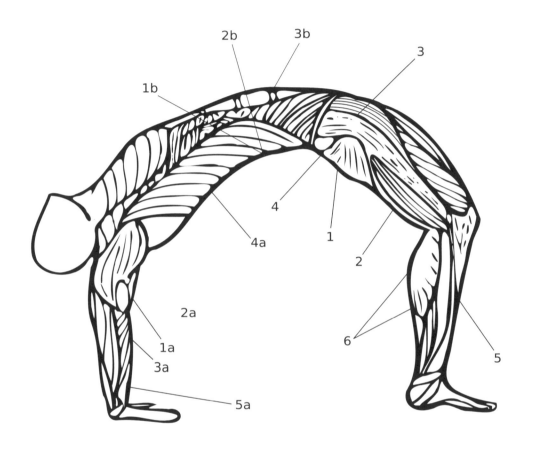

Hip Extensors		
Gluteus maximus	Semitendinosus	Adductor magnus
Gluteus medius	Biceps femoris	Semimembranosus